Pharmaceutical Chemistry and Production: An Introductory Textbook

Authored by

Samir Kumar Mandal

Department of Chemistry,
Saldiha College,
Saldiha, Bankura,
India

&

Rebeca Ghanta

Department of Botany,
Ramananda College,
Bishnupur,
Bankura,
India

Pharmaceutical Chemistry and Production: An Introductory Textbook

Authors: Samir Kumar Mandal and Rebeca Ghanta

ISBN (Online): 978-1-68108-889-1

ISBN (Print): 978-1-68108-890-7

ISBN (Paperback): 978-1-68108-891-4

need for a court order if at any point you breach any terms of this License Agreement. In no event will any delay or failure by Bentham Science Publishers in enforcing your compliance with this License Agreement constitute a waiver of any of its rights.

3. You acknowledge that you have read this License Agreement, and agree to be bound by its terms and conditions. To the extent that any other terms and conditions presented on any website of Bentham Science Publishers conflict with, or are inconsistent with, the terms and conditions set out in this License Agreement, you acknowledge that the terms and conditions set out in this License Agreement shall prevail.

Bentham Science Publishers Ltd.
Executive Suite Y - 2
PO Box 7917, Saif Zone
Sharjah, U.A.E.
Email: subscriptions@benthamscience.net

BENTHAM
SCIENCE

CONTENTS

PREFACE

"Wherever the art of medicine is loved, there is also a love of humanity"
Hippocrates

The main part of this book is pharmaceuticals - what every student of pharmaceutical sciences should know: specially its use, mode of action, chemical synthesis along with the relevant chemistry. Pharmaceuticals are important from top to ground people to survive with care. This necessitates basic understanding about their biological behaviour. This book is looking to outline an approach to pharmaceutical chemistry, at a level easily understood by the beginners. It is written for students of future scientist, and for university/college associates to acquire some basic knowledge in their courses curriculum. The text provides some introductory concepts on drug discovery and drug related terminologies for the beginners. In addition, an introduction to metabolism and synthesis at very basic level to the beginners are presented. Another part contains fermentation that describes its importance mainly in present era, some old protocol, what the convenient processes are, how it can be developed for modern need. Modern technologies at very preliminary level are discussed. Attempts have been taken to provide information of some microbial products. Their natural and commercial production process and development is described in a simple way. It is sincerely hoped that learning about these curriculum will allow students to make informed decisions regarding development of more potent drug and advance production method in their future work.

Attempts have been taken to collect information from different sources and tried best for understanding. In spite of proper care, we undoubtedly believe that there might have error in many reasons. Though the responsibility of the error is sole of us, but constructive suggestions from readers will be appreciated.

We would like to thank my dear students who requested repeatedly to help them in newly implemented CBCS curriculum in India. We are grateful to the authors of books/articles and Institutional reports either through printed manner or web which helped us to prepare the text. We sincerely thank to Bentham Publisher for considering our thought to deliver in the form of book.

We express deep regards to our parents, teachers, well-wishers and special thanks to our little angel 'Suvam' for his natty, sacrifice and support through the entire period of our engagement in preparation of the content. We sincerely miss to share our gratitude to them we lost.

CONSENT FOR PUBLICATION

Not applicable.

CONFLICT OF INTEREST

The authors declare no conflict of interest, financial or otherwise.

ACKNOWLEDGEMENTS

Declared none.

Samir Kumar Mandal
Department of Chemistry
Saldiha College
Saldiha, Bankura
India

&

Rebeca Ghanta
Department of Botany
Ramananda College
Bishnupur, Bankura
India

CHAPTER 1

Drugs and Pharmaceuticals: An Introduction

Abstract: Pharmaceuticals, either natural or synthetic, are important from top to ground people to survive with care. Traditional medicinal plants are the key for the synthetic development of any drugs. Synthesis of an efficient drug depends on the selectivity, affinity, efficiency, metabolic stability, and bioavailability of the compound. This chapter gives very brief idea about Active Ingredient (AI), API, Bactericidal, Bacteriostatic, Binders, Cross-screening, Brand, Generic, Effective Dose Fifty (ED_{50}), Inhibitory Concentration fifty (IC_{50}), Lethal Dose Fifty (LD_{50}), Drug, Medicine, Broad-Spectrum, Narrow-Spectrum, ADME, DMPK, Pharmacodynamics, Pharmacokinetics, Pharmacology, Biopharmaceutical, Pro-Drug, SAR, Synergistic action, *in-vitro, in-vivo* terms to begin freshly.

Keywords: Drug discovery, Pharmaceuticals, Pharmaceutical chemistry, Pharmacology, Pharmacokinetics.

DRUG DISCOVERY

Drug discovery is the process by which new candidate medications are discovered. This process is based on the finding of active ingredients from traditional remedies or by unplanned but fortunate discovery. In ancient India, the use of root to leaf of the "Vasaka" medicinal herb for the treatment of asthma, bronchitis, tuberculosis and others, is well known. Later on, a classical way of pharmacology screened chemical libraries of synthetic small molecules, natural products or extracts in intact cells or whole organisms to identify substances that have a desirable therapeutic effect [1]. In reverse pharmacology, screening of large compounds libraries are useful against isolated biological targets which are hypothesized to be disease-modifying. Results of such screening are then tested in cells and then in animals for efficacy. Though plant-derived natural products were the starting point of new drug design, modern drug design is based on rational design (Fig. **1**) [2 - 7].

Samir Kumar Mandal and Rebeca Ghanta

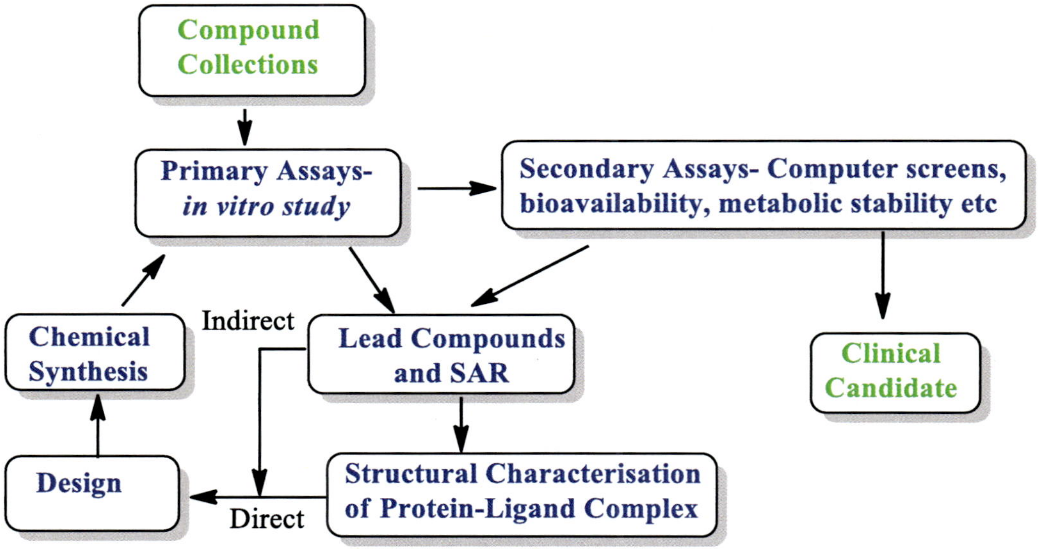

Fig. (1). Drug discovery cycle.

Recently, it has been observed that drug discovery largely depends on the identification of screening hits, medicinal chemistry and optimization of those hits to increase the selectivity, affinity, efficiency, metabolic stability, and bioavailability. If these criteria match, then the process of drug development starts [8]. The best finding is taken for the clinical trial with very expensive Phase I, II and III clinical trials. It takes a lot of time, efforts and money of the pharmaceutical industry to reach the goal. National research laboratory is also involved directly or in collaboration with the pharmaceutical industry. In this partnership, government also grants projects through different funding agencies like DST, UGC, DBT, *etc.* Drug discovery is still a lengthy and inefficient process. Despite advances in technology and understanding of biological systems, this is still expensive and difficult with a low rate of new therapeutic discovery. The approximate cost for research and development of new molecules as a drug is 14 thousand crore INR or 200 crore US Dollar (~2 billion dollar).

IMPORTANT TERMINOLOGY [3-6]

Selectivity

This helps to reduce the potential side effects of a drug.

Affinity

This helps to determine the binding capability with the target.

Efficiency

This helps to find drug efficacy.

Metabolic stability

This helps to increase the half-life of a drug.

Bioavailability

This helps to check its mobility in the biological system.

Cross-screening

This helps to check the off-target activity *i.e.* other than the actual target.

Active Pharmaceutical Ingredient (API)

Active Pharmaceutical Ingredient (API) refers to the biologically active component. This is useful for the formulation of drugs or medicines. Production of API must satisfy the current Good Manufacturing Practices (cGMP).

Drug

A drug is a substance produced naturally or artificially, that is used as an active ingredient of medicine in the diagnosis, mitigation, treatment, or prevention of a disease or relief of uneasiness. It could have harmful side effects or positive effects. Generally, a drug is most commonly a small organic molecule that activates or inhibits the function of a biomolecule such as a protein, which in turn results in a therapeutic benefit to the organism—for example, ibuprofen, paracetamol, sulfacetamide, *etc.*

Medicine

Medicine is an external substance that is administered to ease suffering. Medication is apparently used for a specific therapeutic purpose. It does not have to be manufactured, it may be extracted from the living system. A medicine may contain other substances other than active ingredients (AI) that assist the formulation and increase efficacy.

The bottom-line, ***all medicines are drugs, but all drugs are not medicines***.

Biopharmaceutical

A pharmaceutical is a substance that is extracted from, or semi synthesized from biological sources like humans, animals, or microorganisms. This is produced using biotechnology. They are sugars, proteins, nucleic acids, living cells, or tissues used for therapeutic or *in vivo* diagnostic purposes. Chemically synthesized small organic molecule is a drug but not a biopharmaceutical for this reason. For example, recombinant human insulin (rHI, trade name Humulin) was the first biopharmaceutical approved for therapeutic use. This was developed by Genentech and marketed by Eli Lily in 1982.

Pro-Drug

A compound is said to be a prodrug if, after administration, it undergoes metabolism (*i.e.*, converted within the body) into a pharmacologically active drug. For example, aspirin is a prodrug, which is transformed into salicylate in the stomach, which is responsible for analgesic effects.

Brand Name Drug

The brand name is the name of a drug that has a trade name and is protected by a patent [3, 5]. This can be produced and sold only by the company holding the patent. For example, Nurofen® is the brand name of ibuprofen given by Reckitt Benckiser Healthcare [9]. Brand names are usually capitalized while generic names are not.

Generic Drug

A drug that has the same chemical substance as the drug that is developed initially patented and innovated. Generics only become available after the patent expires on a brand name drug. For example, McNeil Consumer Healthcare's Tylenol® is the brand name of generic drug acetaminophen [9]. Brand names are usually capitalized words and ended with® while generic names are not [3, 5].

Pharmacodynamics (PD)

Pharmacodynamics [3] is the study of the biochemical and physiological effects of drugs [3]. It gives information of the molecular action of a drug on its target and deals with receptors, ion channels, enzymes, immune system. Thus pharmacodynamics deals with the mechanism of a drug on the body.

Pharmacokinetics (PK)

Pharmacokinetics is the study of the fate of substances administered to a living organism [3]. It gives the information of ADME (**A**bsorption, **D**istribution, **M**etabolism, and **E**limination) properties of the drug [3, 5]. Thus pharmacokinetics deals with the movement of drugs within the body.

ADME (**A**bsorption, **D**istribution, **M**etabolism, and **E**limination) gives the idea of

- Absorption: This tells about the bioavailability rate in a living system
- Distribution: This tells about the place where the drug is distributed
- Metabolism: This tells about the metabolite formed in the body - whether they are active or toxic
- Elimination: This tells about the route of elimination of the drug from the body

DMPK (**D**rug **M**etabolism and **P**harmaco-**K**inetics)

This is an important part of studying **ADME** (**A**bsorption, **D**istribution, **M**etabolism, and **E**limination) properties in drug design and screening.

Lethal Dose Fifty (LD_{50})

LD stands for "Lethal Dose". LD_{50} is the amount of a substance, given all at once, which causes the death of 50% (one half) of a group of test living systems *i.e.* animals [3]. The LD_{50} is one way to measure the short-term poisoning potential (acute toxicity) of a material.

Effective Dose Fifty (ED_{50})

ED stands for "Effective Dose". ED_{50} is the amount of a substance, given all at once, which produces a therapeutic response or desired effect in 50% of the population [3]. The ED_{50} is one way to measure the effective short-term potential of a material.

Inhibitory Concentration Fifty (IC_{50})

IC stands for "Inhibitory Concentration". This refers to the concentration of an inhibitor where the response (or binding) is reduced by half (50%) [3]. Though it is very simple but to determine these values, there are several complexities and ambiguities. The lower the IC_{50} of the drug molecule, the more potent it is considered.

Pharmaceutical Formulation

It is the process in which the active pharmaceutical ingredients, including other chemical substances are combined to produce a final dose [3, 5]. Other substances are inactive ingredients that are required to formulate the final dose form of the drug. They are fillers, disintegrants, lubricants, glidants, and binders and may be water, co-solvents, buffering agents, and pH-adjusting agents [10]. Generally, a formulation is of two types: enteral formulation in the form of capsules, tablets, and pills and parenteral formulation in the form of injections. Formulation depends on the particle size, polymorphism, pH, stability and solubility of a drug as these factors affect the physico-chemical properties and the bioavailability of the drug [11]. For example, if a drug needs to absorb quickly, then tablet form is preferable, while for little delayed absorption, capsule form is preferable. Pills are generally coated with sugar, varnish, wax and others to mask the taste of the dose. However, there are many techniques that can sustain the release of drugs either in tablet or capsule form.

In vivo and *in vitro* Study

These two common terms are used in drug design and development. Before launching the drug in the market, it is studied in the laboratory first to check if the drug is active or not (***in vitro*** **study**). If the drug is active, then it is applied into the living system (***in vivo*** **study**) to check that the drug is working fine or not. The easiest way to remember the difference is that activity study *in vivo* that means inside the living organism and *in vitro* means outside the living organism [5].

Synergistic Action

If the drugs work together, so the total effect is greater than the sum of the two, then the action is said to be synergistic action [3, 5]. Some drugs work better when used in combination. For example, individually, carbon tetrachloride and ethyl alcohol are toxic to the liver but when they are together, they cause more injury than the sum of their effect. Similarly, sulfamethoxazole shows synergistic action when used in combination with trimethoprim.

Antibiotic Drug

A drug is said to be an antibiotic if it kills or slows the growth of bacteria. It cures infectious diseases caused by bacteria [3]. Pathogenic bacteria cause disease when they are able to gain access to vulnerable parts of the living system and multiply rapidly, making substantial injury in the body. Antibiotics fall in the class of antimicrobials, a larger group that also include anti-virals, anti-fungals, and antiparasitic drugs. Antibiotics are chemicals produced by or derived from microorganisms (*i.e.* bacteria and fungi). The first antibiotic, penicillin, was discovered by Alexander Fleming in 1928.

Though both the term antibiotics and antibacterials are used synonymously, antibacterial substances only work against the bacteria and these antibacterial compounds, rather killing those harmful bacteria, help to slow down their activities. So, all antibiotics are antibacterial, but all antibacterials are not antibiotics'.

There are different modes of action of antibiotics. Antibiotics, like penicillin, block specific enzymes. Peptide-based antibiotics often form complexes with metal ions and upset the control of ion permeability in bacterial membranes. Some of the polyene antibiotics interfere with proton and ion transport in fungal membranes. Tetracyclines and many other antibiotics interfere directly with protein synthesis. In many cases, they intercalate into DNA molecules like benzene.

Bactericidal Antibiotics

Antibiotics that work by killing bacteria are called bactericidal antibiotics [5]. Bacteriostatic antibiotics inhibit cell wall synthesis—for example, cephalosporins, daptomycin, fluoroquinolones, metronidazole, co-trimoxazole, dapsone, nalidixic acid, *etc.*

Bacteriostatic Antibiotics

Antibiotics that work by stopping the reproduction or growth of bacteria are called bacteriostatic antibiotics [5]. Bacteriostatic antibiotics stop reproduction by interfering DNA replication and growth by inhibiting bacterial protein synthesis, for example, tetracyclines, sulfacetamide, co-trimoxazole, dapsone, nalidixic acid, *etc.*

It is very difficult to say, which is more effective between bacteriostatic antibiotics and bactericidal antibiotics. However, high concentrations of some bacteriostatic agents are bactericidal.

Broad-Spectrum Antibiotics

Antibiotics that can be used to treat a wide range of infections are called ***broad-spectrum*** antibiotics [5]. They are used when a bacterial infection is suspected but of an unknown group. This is risky as they may develop resistance to bacteria; for example, ampicillin, tetracycline, chloramphenicol, trimethoprim, *etc.*

Narrow-Spectrum Antibiotics

Antibiotics that can be used to treat specific types of bacteria are called ***narrow-spectrum*** antibiotics [5]. These antibiotics are used for the specific infection when the organism is known. They does not kill many of the normal microorganisms in the body as the broad-spectrum antibiotics do. Their use is little risky as they develop less resistance to bacteria. For example, penicillin G is very effective at killing gram-positive bacteria but not very effective against gram-negative bacteria.

Antibiotic Resistance

Bacteria are said to be antibiotic-resistant if not killed by a certain drug [3]. Repeated use of a drug for bacteria can lead to development of resistance, by changing their structure, which makes the drug ineffective. This is now a serious issue in medical science. For example, penicillin is resistant to *Staphylococcus aureus*, and daptomycin is resistant to *staphylococcus aureus.*

Antiviral Drugs

Antiviral drugs are a class of medication used for treating viral infections [5]. This class of drugs inhibits viral entry, uncoating, nucleic acid biosynthesis and prevents viral escape from endosomes, and viral release from infected cells. It is hard to target viruses because human viruses replicate inside human cells. Most antivirals are target specific viruses, while a broad-spectrum antiviral is effective against a wide range of viruses. Unlike most antibiotics, antiviral drugs do not destroy their target pathogen; instead, they inhibit their development. For example, acyclovir is an antiviral agent used to treat chickenpox.

Antifungal Drugs

The drugs that interfere with ergosterol synthesis bind to ergosterol to disrupt fungal cell membrane integrity, or target cell wall-specific components or other cellular proteins called antifungal drugs [5]. For example, fluconazole, a triazole derivative, acts as an antifungal agent by *inhibiting cell wall synthesis.*

DESIGN AND DEVELOPMENT

Any functional disorder in a particular metabolic or signaling pathway of the living system by a bio-molecule, e.g. protein or nucleic acid, is associated with a specific disease condition or pathology or the infectivity or survival of a microbial pathogen. In some cases, small molecules are designed to inhibit or enhance the activity of such functions in the specific disease [11-16]. A small molecule is designed such that it is complementary in shape and charge to the bio-molecular target binding site.

This is very crucial since the small molecule must not interact with the off-target to avoid side effects. Thus a small organic molecule becomes a drug if it is designed and synthesized chemically or isolated from a biological system to inhibit or enhance the activity of target function in the specific disease. Small molecule drugs are designed and synthesized chemically but biopolymer-based drugs produced through biological processes are becoming increasingly more common. When a lead compound is selected for the target, it is developed by chemists to improve certain features by using structure-activity-relationship (SAR) [2, 3-6].

In general, drugs work by interacting with receptors on the surface of cells or enzymes within cells [3-7, 13-14]. Receptor and enzyme molecules allow the substances that can fit precisely to attach with them. This is generally known as the lock and key model. While drug binds with the target receptor site, they can act in two ways. Either they block the physiological function of the protein or mimicits effect. There are some natural molecules, usually called agonists, that bind with protein and cause to response in different issues; these are morphine, nicotine, phenylephrine, and isoproterenol. Drug molecules can also act as an agonist. The drug molecules that interact selectively with receptors but do not lead to an observed effect are called antagonists. In that case, they reduce the action of an agonist at the receptor site involved. In other cases, drugs target the enzymes and are considered as inhibitors or activators. Aspirin, COX-2 inhibitors and HIV protease inhibitors are common examples in this case.

Most common nonsteroidal anti-inflammatory drugs (NSAID) work by inhibiting the cyclooxygenase pathway [13, 14]. This process starts with arachidonic acid and is converted by the enzyme cyclooxygenase to synthesize different prostaglandins. The prostaglandins stimulate many regulatory functions and responses in the body, including inflammation and increased sensitivity to pain. Cyclooxygenase (COX-1) is located in the stomach wall and regulated by NSAIDs.

OUTLINES OF DRUG DEVELOPMENT PROCESS [6].

Discovery, Screening and R&D [about 5-6 yrs]	• Potential therapeutic targets are identified based on the studies of the physiological, cellular, genetic basis of disease. • New compounds are isolated and purified from natural sources or synthesized. • Now, *in vitro,* assays are developed to measure the effect of potential therapeutics. • Based on the *in vitro* assay, 5,000-10,000 new and previously developed compounds are tested to ensure the biological activity. • Almost 250 of the compounds tested having the desired activities are considered as "hits".
FDA Review [about 1-2 months]	• Improved "hits" are known as "lead compounds". Satisfactory "hits" are chosen for chemical modification in order to improve target specificity, potency, chemical and metabolic stability, water-solubility, including other pharmacological parameters. • For safety and efficacy, *in vivo* experiment is done with the lead compounds on animals such as mice and rats. • An Investigational New Drug Application (NDA) is filed with the FDA (Food and Drug Administration) before the preclinical study.
Develop and Monitoring [about 6-8 yrs]	• **Phase I** clinical trials consist of drug safety studies in healthy humans (about 1 year). • **Phase II** clinical trials test whether a drug works in a small number of patients affected by the disease (about 2 years). • **Phase III** clinical trials test on large numbers of patients (about 3 years).
FDA Review	• A New Drug Application (NDA) is filed with the FDA (about 1.5-2.5 years). • This involves FDA evaluation and submission
Drug Launch / Marketing	• Administrative clearance • Planning for marketing with best understanding with physicians, patients, and payers • Clinical data and success report

Generally, the new drug development process is a tedious process and takes 12-15 years [6, 8, 11-12]. In the beginning, a long term interaction between theoretical biology and medicinal chemistry takes place to determine a compound's biological activity in the body and optimize the compound. With the satisfaction of human studies, clinical observations are important to test hypotheses about how a candidate drug may target cells. Safety and effective doses are considered sincerely and compared for their ability relative to standard therapy. This complex process is based on several steps ranging from initial target detection and validation, through assay development, high output relative to input screening, hit identification, and lead optimization to the selection of a candidate molecule for clinical development [8]. Different funding agencies from national levels are assisting in the development of the new drug. In India, time to time approval is needed from the Indian Council of Medical Research (ICMR) and Drugs Controller General of India (DCGI) for regulatory permissions for the conduct of clinical trials. However, DCGI is advised by the Drug Consultative Committee (DCC) and the Drug Technical Advisory Board (DTAB). In the US, the funding agency is the National Institutes of Health (NIH) and in India, the funding agencies are the Indian Council of Medical Research (ICMR), Department of Biotechnology (DBT), Council of Scientific and Industrial Research (CSIR).

NOMENCLATURE OF DRUGS

The chemists prefer to name a drug based on its chemical structure. This becomes unsuitable for a doctor to remember the name all the time while prescribing a drug. However the manufacturing companies make it commercial and give their brand name.

Thus any drug may have names in all three of the following classes [3, 15]:

1. Chemical name

The full chemical name based on the chemical structure.

2. Non-proprietary Name

A generic (non-proprietary) name is used in pharmacopeias and chosen by official bodies.

3. Proprietary Name

A brand (proprietary) name is the name given by a pharmaceutical company.

For example, the generic name of diazepam is benzodiazepine. Zepose® is the brand name of diazepam, marketed by Cipla.

Chemical name: benzodiazepine
Non-proprietary Name: diazepam
Proprietary Name: Zepose® (Cipla), Valium® (Ahaan Healthcare), Placidox® (Lupin), Prazep® (Sun)

Either structural information or the activity is often considered for naming a drug [9]. This helps to identify the name with the suffix. For example, drug names with suffix –olol are adrenoceptor (beta) blockers, while –pril are angiotensin-converting enzyme (ACE) inhibitors. A very common drug name with suffix –floxacin, is quinolone antimicrobials. Pharmaceutical companies have the liberty to manufacture a well-established drug without any patent restriction. But they must follow official pharmacopoeial quality criteria to the regulatory authority for a license to market the drug.

CLASSIFICATION OF DRUGS

There is no uniform system for classifying the drugs that addresses all the issues. This is because of the different view of chemists, pharmacologists, doctors and other associates [5]. They are generally classified as:

1. **Body system**

   Drugs classified according to the organ or system on which they act *e.g.*, alimentary, cardiovascular, dermatological, nervous system, and respiratory system.

2. **Therapeutic use**

   Drugs classified according to the pathology they are used to treat *e.g.* receptor blockers, enzyme inhibitors, carrier molecules, and ion channels.

3. **Mode or Site of Action**

   Drugs are classified according to the anatomical changes or functional changes at the cellular level resulting from the exposure of a living organism to a substance.

- Molecular interaction, *e.g.* glucoside, alkaloid, steroid
- Cellular site, *e.g.* loop diuretic, catecholamine uptake inhibitor

4. **Molecular Structure**

   Drugs that are classified according to the chemical structure include, glycoside, alkaloid, and steroid.

Very common types of drugs are antibiotics, antifungals *etc.* Their classifications are given below.

CLASSIFICATION

Antibiotic Drugs

Based on the structures, antibiotics are mainly classified into six major classes [5]:

- ***Beta-Lactams***: Penicillins, Amoxicillin, Cephalosporins, monobactams, carbapenems and carbacephems
- ***Macrolides***: Clarithromycin, Azithromycin, Fidaxomicin, Erythromycin
- ***Fluoroquinolones***: Norfloxacin, Moxifloxacin, Ciprofloxacin
- ***Sulfonamides***: Co-trimoxazole, trimethoprim
- ***Tetracyclines***: Doxycycline, Minocycline, Oxytetracycline, Tetracycline
- ***Aminoglycosides***: Gentamicin, Amikacin, Tobramycin, Neomycin, Strepto-mycin

Antifungal Drugs

They are classified based on treatment, chemical structure and mechanism of action [5].

A. Classification Based on Treatment

*1. **Drugs for Systemic Fungal Infections***

Polyene Antibiotics: Amphotericin B

Pyrimidine Antimetabolites: Flucytosine

Antifungal Azoles: Ketoconazole, Fluconazole, Itraconazole, Voriconazole

Echinocandins: Caspofungin, Micafungin, and Anidulafungin

*2. **Drugs for Superficial Fungal Infections:*** Griseofulvin, Iodide

*3. **Topical drugs:***

Polyene Antibiotics: Nystatin, Hamycin, Natamycin

Azoles :Miconazole, Econazole, Clotrimazole

Organic Acids and Salt: Benzoic acid, Sodium thiosulfate

B. Based on the Mechanism of Action

1. Inhibit Ergosterol Synthesis: Imidazoles subclass include ketoconazole, econazole, miconazole, clotrimazole, and oxiconazole; triazoles subclass include fluconazole, itoconazole, and posaconazole; allylamines subclass include terbinafine, and naftifine.

2. Bind Ergosterol for Disruption of Cell Membrane: Polyenes class include Nystatin, Amphotericin-B

3. Inhibit Cell Wall Synthesis: Echinocandins, Caspofungin, Pneumocandins

4. Inhibition of Nucleic Acid Synthesis: Flucytocine, Griseofulvin

C. Based on the chemical structure

1. *Polyenes*: These bind ergosterol in the cell membrane and create pores that disrupt the membrane. For example, Nystatin, Amphotericin-B, *etc.*

2. *Azoles*: These inhibit lanosterol 14-α-demethylase enzyme, required to convert lanosterol into ergosterol. Imidazoles subclass include ketoconazole, econazole, miconazole, clotrimazole, and oxiconazole; triazoles subclass include fluconazole, itraconazole, and posaconazole.

3. *Allylamines*: These inhibit squalene epoxidase. These are allylamine derivative antifungals; for example, terbinafine, naftifine, *etc.*

4. *Pyrimidine*: These inhibit nucleic acid synthesis. These are pyrimidine antifungals; for example, flucytocine.

5. *Echinocandins*: This inhibits the synthesis of glucan in the cell wall via the enzyme 1,3-β-glucan synthase. These are peptide antifungals; for example, caspofungin, micafungin, and anidulafungin.

CHAPTER 2

Analgesics, Antipyretic and Anti-Inflammatory Drugs

Abstract: This chapter deals with the brand names, uses, mode of action and side effects of analgesics, antipyretic and anti-inflammatory drugs *e.g.* aspirin, paracetamol and ibuprofen. A brief history of their discovery has also been discussed in this chapter. Various synthetic methods have shown here along with the relevant chemistry. This involves industrial method, green technology and asymmetric synthesis.

Keywords: Drug discovery, Pharmaceuticals, Pharmaceutical chemistry, Pharmacology, Pharmacokinetics.

ANALGESICS AND ANTI-INFLAMMATORY DRUGS

Aspirin

The bark and leaves of willow trees have been used as a pain killer for a long time. The active component of the bark and leaves of willow trees is salicylic acid (SA), which creates pH~2.9-3.0 in the body. Salicylic acid is extremely bitter in taste, and its frequent use can cause severe stomach irritation. This pH is higher than stomach pH~4.0; as a result, it causes disturbance in the stomach [16]. In comparison, the monoprotic acetylsalicylic acid (ASA, aspirin) is less acidic (pKa = 4.57) as an ester is replaced with the acidic phenol in ASA. ASA is less soluble in water, but its Na-salt is soluble. Thus increased acidity in the body causes deposition of ASA. The search for a milder form of this pain reliever (analgesics) led to the successful synthesis of acetylsalicylic acid by the German chemist Felix Hoffmann in 1893. It has weak antipyretic properties. It is also used synthetically for the preparation of salbutamol, an anti-asthma drug, using Friedel–Crafts acylation as one of the key steps.

Samir Kumar Mandal and Rebeca Ghanta

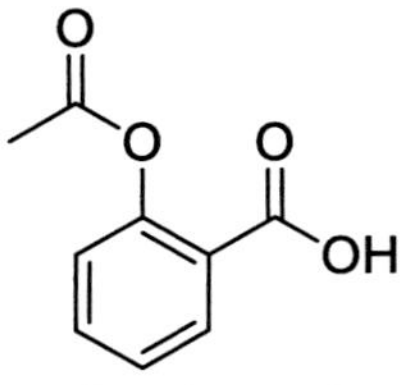

2-acetoxybenzoic acid
(Aspirin)

It is used as a fever reducer, pain reliever and has antiplatelet effects [3, 5-7]. It is usually taken once a day to lower the risk of a heart attack or stroke for its anti-blood clotting effect. A typical dosage ranges from 50 milligrams (mg) to 6,000 mg daily. Use of aspirin may cause easy bruising, bleeding, difficulty in hearing, ringing in the ears, kidney problems, persistent or severe nausea, vomiting, unexplained tiredness, dizziness, dark urine, yellowing eyes or skin. Long-term use of aspirin irreversibly blocks the formation of thromboxane A2 in platelets that results in an inhibitory effect on platelet aggregation [13, 14]. It is common with drugs in the pill form; the commercial preparations often contain other ingredients such as binders and fillers, which help to form pills that do not fall apart under normal storage and transport. The amount of ASA that should be contained in a tablet differs from brand to brand and is indicated on the package.

In Inflammation and pain are reduced by inhibiting the synthesis of prostaglandin (PG) and thromboxanes *via* irreversible (reversible for ibuprofen) inactivation of the cyclooxygenase (COX) enzyme. This is due to the acetylation of the amine group of a serine residue in the COX enzyme by aspirin. Contrary to this, it may cause the ulcer in the stomatch as prostaglandin controls the acid secretion in the body [7, 13].

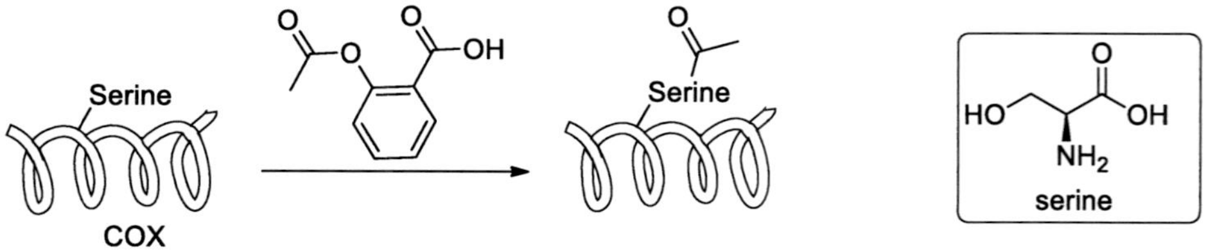

Synthetic Use of Aspirin

Aspirin is used in the production of salbutamol [3, 16], which is used to relieve symptoms of asthma. Salbutamol works by relaxing the muscles of the airways into the lungs, making it easier to breathe.

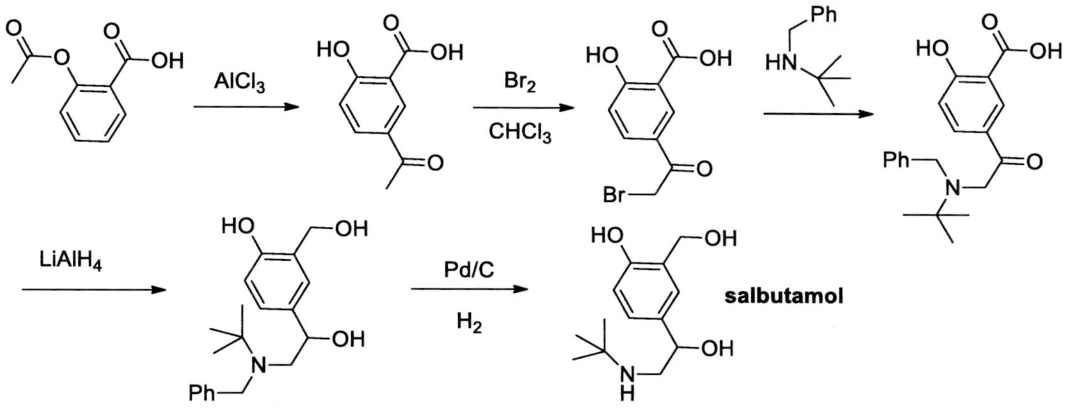

Acetylation Method

ASA is synthesized from salicylic acid *via* esterification reaction and the salicylic acid is prepared industrially *via* Kolbe–Schmitt process. In the first steps, a suspension of salicylic acid in excess of acetic anhydride is made. Acetic anhydride serves as both a reactant and a solvent. A catalyst is required for this reaction. Phosphoric acid, H_3PO_4, is usually used as a catalyst; others include H_2SO_4, $MgBr_2.OEt_2$, $AlCl_3$, $CaCO_3$, NaOAc, NEt_3, and 4-N, N-dimethylaminopyridine (DMAP) [16, 17]. As the reaction proceeds, the solid salicylic acid disappears and the acetylsalicylic acid product remains dissolved in the hot solution. Once all solid disappears, the reaction is completed, and the presence of salicylic acid may be tested with $FeCl_3$ solution by taking an aliquot of the reaction. Acetic anhydride is very reactive toward water, so the hydrolysis must be done slowly with drop-wise addition of water for this purpose. After this, more water is added and the flask is placed in an ice bath to lower the solubility and precipitate the ASA product. The product is then collected by filtration.

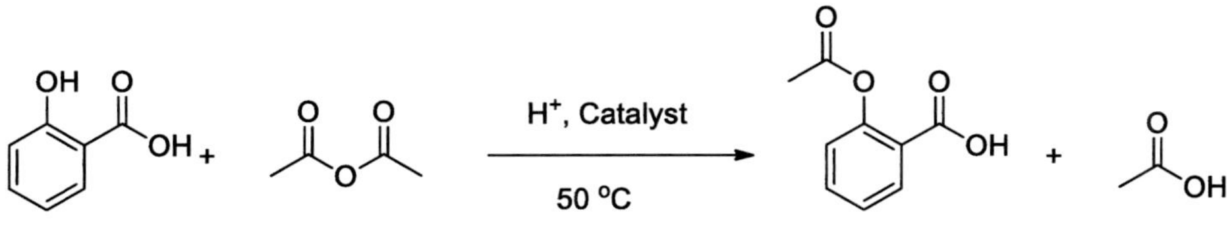

The same process is carried out in a greener way under MW irradiation to eliminate the reaction time and the conventional heating process [16c]. There are many approaches where solvent and catalyst-free MW irradiation reaction conditions are reported in high yielding. One of the main reasons for not using the catalyst under MW condition is the increase in the polarity of the media or charge separation in the reaction transition state (the catalyst increases the polarity of the molecules undergoing reaction in the conventional process), which allows a faster reaction under microwave irradiation.

Ibuprofen

Ibuprofen is considered a non-steroidal anti-inflammatory drug (NSAID) [7]. The formula of ibuprofen is 2-(4-isobutylphenyl) propionic acid, marketed as Nurofen®. It was initially developed in 1960 during research for a safer alternative for aspirin. These drugs are used for the management of mild to moderate pain, fever, and inflammation. Ibuprofen blocks the enzyme (cyclooxygenase) that makes prostaglandins, resulting in lower levels of prostaglandins that are responsible for pain and fever. As a consequence, the use of Ibuprofen reduces inflammation, pain and fever. It was first used against rheumatoid arthritis in the UK in 1969 and in the USA in 1974.

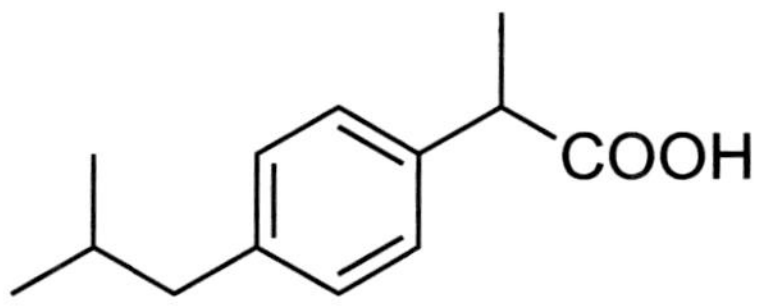

2-(4-isobutylphenyl)propanoic acid

(Ibuprofen)

Ibuprofen may cause rashes, ringing in the ears, headaches, dizziness, drowsiness, abdominal pain, nausea, diarrhea, constipation, and heartburn. As a member of NSAIDs, ibuprofen may reduce the ability of blood to clot and therefore increase bleeding after an injury. The most serious issues are that ibuprofen may cause ulceration of the stomach or intestine, and the ulcers may bleed. For minor issues like aches, mild to moderate pain, menstrual cramps, and fever, the usual adult dose is 200 or 400 mg every 4 to 6 hours [13, 14]. Arthritis is treated with 300 to 800 mg 3 or 4 times daily.

The name ibuprofen is a combination of three units, namely, ibu (isobutyl), pro (propyl), fen (phenyl). The S-enantiomer is believed to be the more pharmacologically active enantiomer. Ibuprofen is administered as a racemic mixture. Once administered, the R-enantiomer undergoes interconversion to the S-enantiomer *in vivo* by the activity of the alpha-methylacyl-CoA racemase enzyme *i.e.* racimised in the body. So the effect of R-isomer (may be considered as prodrug) is minimized *in vivo*, allowing its easy availability due to the low production cost of the racemic compound [7, 13].

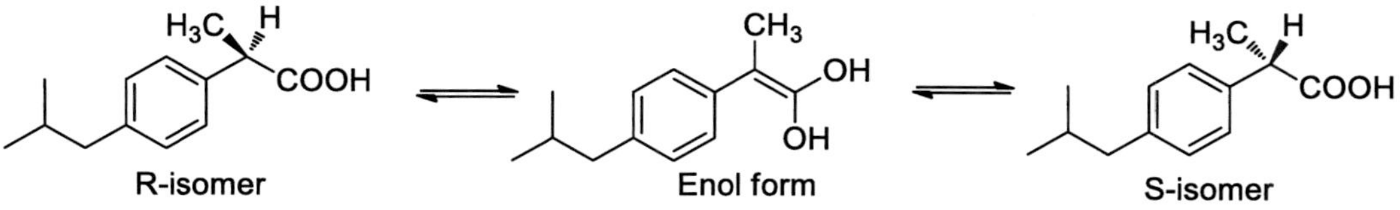

Synthesis

Boot Method

This is one of the most popular ways to formulate ibuprofen. This older commercial process was developed by the Boot Pure Drug Company [7]. Synthesis of ibuprofen starts with isobutylbenzene and uses Friedel-Crafts acylation. This process involves 6 steps to produce ibuprofen *via* Darzens reaction.

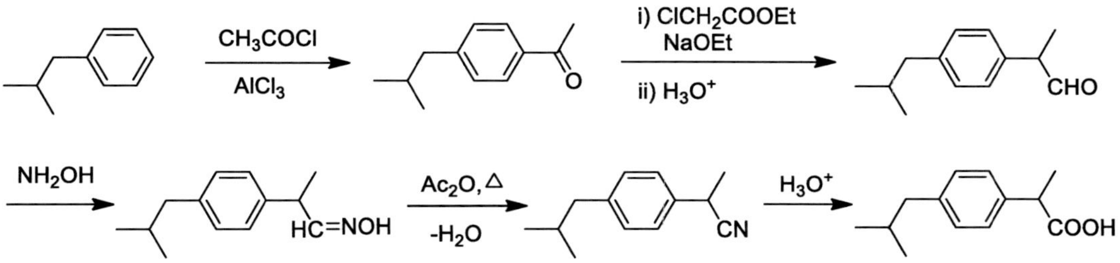

Hoechst–Celanese Methods

Hoechst is also a popular way to formulate ibuprofen. This newer commercial process was developed by the Hoechst Company. Synthesis of ibuprofen starts with isobutylbenzene based on Friedel-Crafts acylation. Hoesch process used the palladium catalyst (for hydrogenation and Carbonylation) and completed the synthesis of ibuprofen in 3 steps. This process is considered as the greener synthesis of ibuprofen as it reduces the use of a huge amount of solvent in the Boot process.

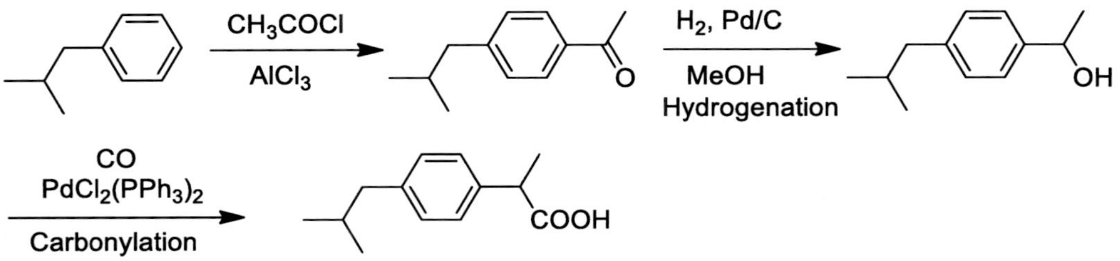

Schlosser Method

Metalation of the aromatic compound is of two types-a) ortho-metalation directed by the group present in the ring and b) side chain metalation at benzylic position [18b]. Consecutive metalation at the benzylic position and electrophilic substitution of p-xylene in three steps provide ibuprofen with moderate yield. The electrophilic substitution is a crucial step here as it results in sequentially correct order.

Directed Ortho Metalation

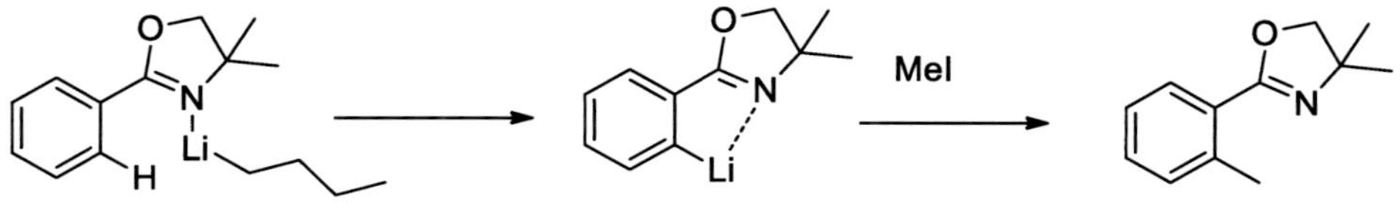

Benzylic Metalation

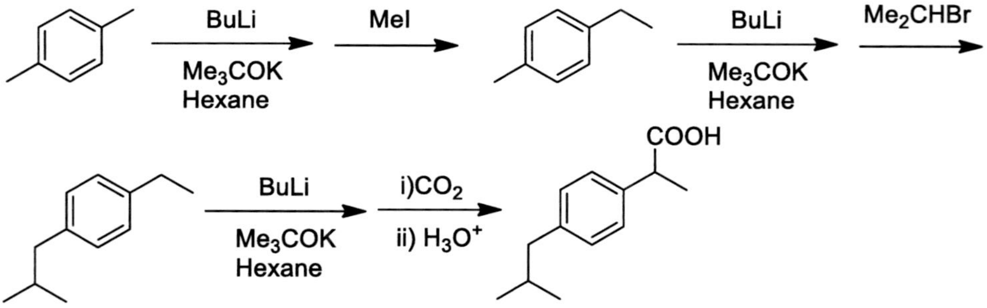

Green Synthesis

Daniel J. Swartling has claimed a sustainable synthesis of ibuprofen using solar energy as an alternative source of energy [18a, 18c]. In this process, no electrical heating is necessary but the synthesis is carried out through solar energy using a parabolic mirror as a solar reflector. This synthesis involves Friedel-Craft acylation and Wolff–Kishner reduction followed by Grignard addition.

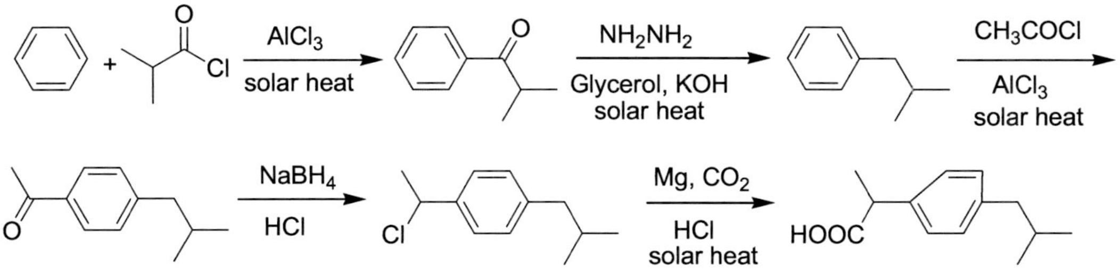

Asymmetric Synthesis

Asymmetric synthesis of ibuprofen is conducted by Aspergillus niger [18d]. Aspergillus niger LCP 521 hydrolyses the racemic epoxide to give the (R)-diol. Unreacted (S)-epoxide is separated by solvent extraction. The chiral (S)-epoxide on hydrogenolysis with Pd/C and H_2 in DMF results in (S)-alcohol followed by oxidation with $KMnO_4$ and sulfuric acid which gives the desired (S)-ibuprofen. The hydrolyzed diol is recycled to racemic epoxide by reaction with HBr in acetic acid followed by cyclization of the intermediate bromohydrin with KOH.

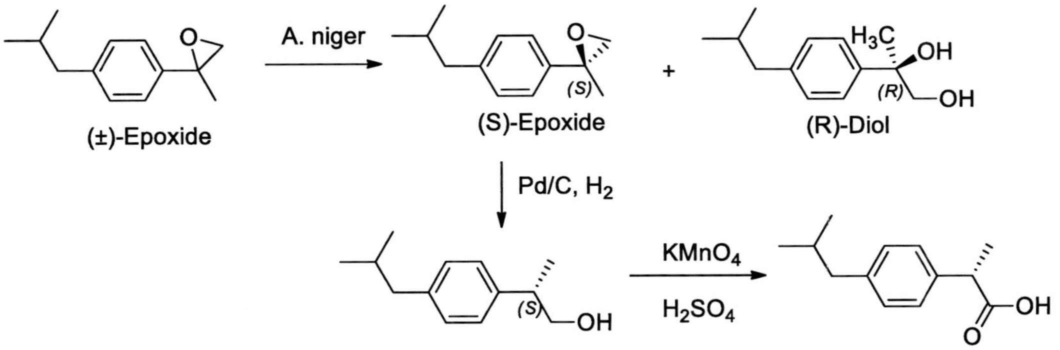

ANALGESICS AND ANTIPYRETICS DRUGS

Paracetamol

Paracetamol is considered as analgesics (pain relievers) and antipyretics (fever reducers) drug [19a]. It is also known as acetaminophen or N-acetyl-para-aminophenol (APAP) and is used to treat mild to moderate pain such as headaches, menstrual periods, toothaches, migraine, nerve pain, backaches, sore throat, muscle aches, osteoarthritis *etc*., though most of us know it as a drug for fever. When cinchona tree (active ingredient quinine, which is an anti-fever agent but mostly used for the treatment of malaria) became scarce, people started looking for other alternatives of antipyretic agents and used phenacetin. Accidentally paracetamol was discovered in the urine of individuals who had taken phenacetin in 1893. In 1948, the analgesic effect of paracetamol was established. Paracetamol was first marketed in the United States in 1950 under the name Triagesic, a combination of paracetamol, aspirin, and caffeine. Paracetamol was first synthesized in 1878 by Harmon Northrop Morse *via* the reduction of *para*-nitrophenol with tin in glacial acetic acid.

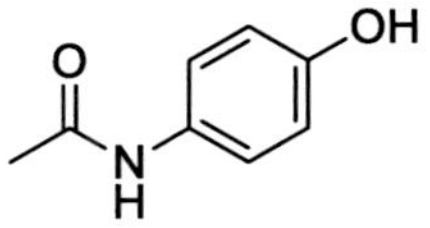

N-(4-hydroxyphenyl)acetamide
(Acetaminophen)

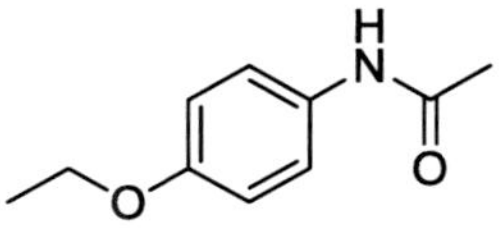

Phenaacetin

Paracetamol works by blocking chemical messengers in the brain that tell us we are suffering from pain. It reduces the production of prostaglandins; unlike aspirin, paracetamol does not have much anti-inflammatory action. It reduces the oxidized form of the COX enzyme (cyclooxygenase), preventing it from forming pro-inflammatory chemicals. This is often used after surgery in most of the cases. The medicine is effective in a body for 4-6 hours. So the next dose is suggested with every 5-6 hours interval. This medicine is not recommended for use in pregnant women though it may be used during breast feeding. In any case, it is better to consult the doctor. Its overdose is severely dangerous and may result in liver damage with ultimate death. Paracetamol is metabolized into a harmful oxidizing agent, N-hydroxyl amine compound and this destroys the glutathione. At a normal dose, everything remains normal as long as there are sufficient glutathiones present [13, 14]. Once excess paracetamol is used, glutathione reacts with the metabolite of paracetamol irreversibly and permanent damage occurs. So it is not advised to the patients with liver diseases to take medicine without consultation of a doctor and also to patients suffering from malnourishment due to the increased risk of severe adverse effects.

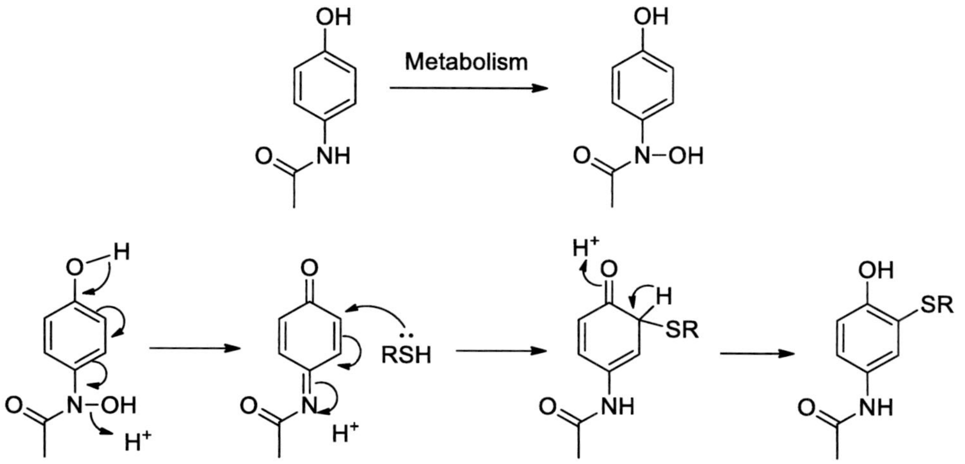

Synthesis

Boot Methods

Phenol on nitration produces two isomers, from which, 4-nitrophenol is separated by steam distillation. *Ortho*-isomer is more steam volatile for intermolecular hydrogen bonds and is steam distilled easily to get *para*-isomer. Then it is reduced to aminophenol, using sodium borohydride followed by chemoselective acetylation with one equivalent of acetic anhydride in pyridine to form N-acetyl-para-aminophenol, suggesting aromatic amine group to be more nucleophilic compared to the phenolic-OH group. Excess acetic anhydride in toluene at 100 °C acetylated both amine and phenol group [19c].

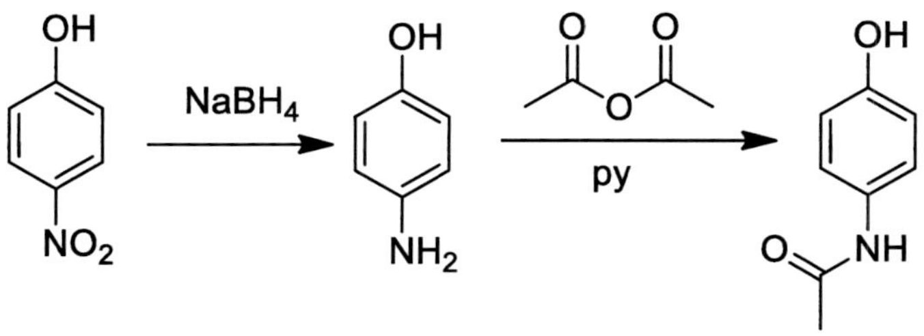

Alternatively, the double acetylated product of para-aminophenol is easily hydrolysed to paracetamol. This is observed due to the higher reactivity of ester compared to amide bond in the presence of aqueous sodium hydroxide.

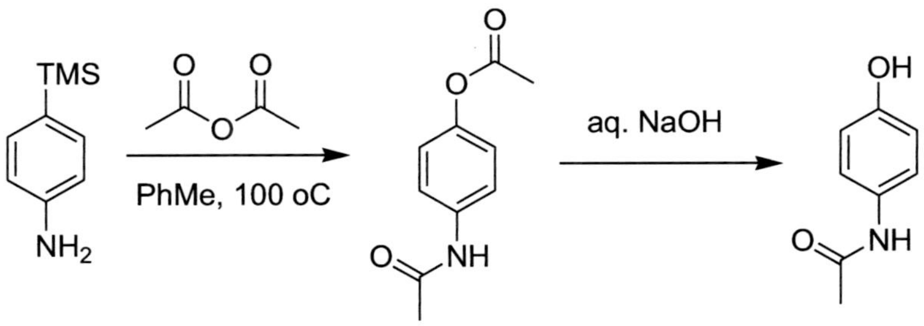

<u>Hoechst–Celanese Methods</u>

This method involves HF catalysed acetylation of phenol with acetic anhydride followed by Beckmann rearrangement of the ketoxime formed from the para-hydroxyacetophenone and hydroxylamine hydrochloride [19d]. This process is greener than the Boot method.

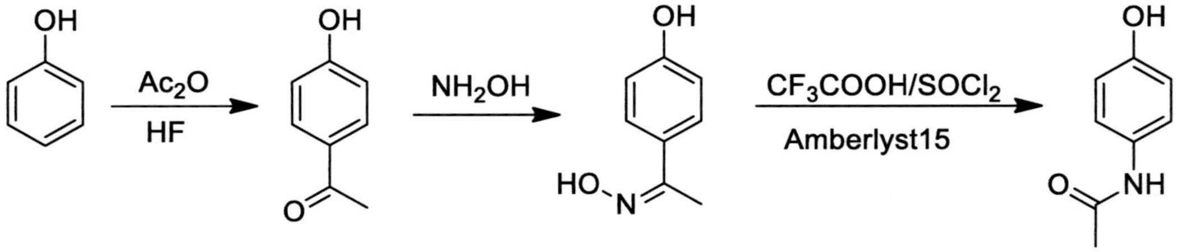

<u>Green Synthesis</u>

Very recently, M. Lemaire uses ammonium acetate as an amidating agent for selective and high yielding one step synthesis of paracetamol from hydroquinone [19b]. The process involves a multigram scale in acetic acid media at elevated temperature. The solvent and the byproducts are easily recycled in this process.

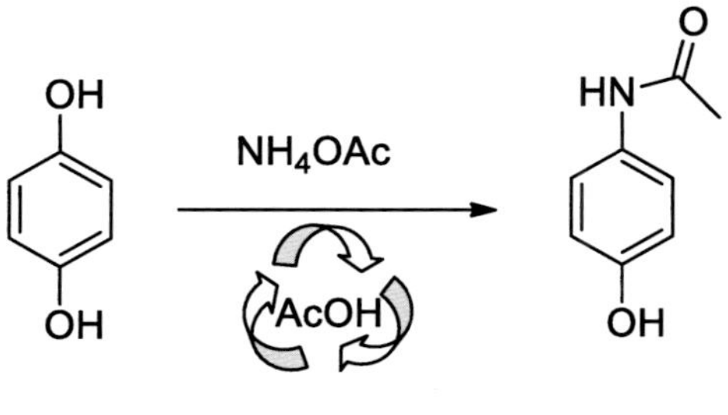

CHAPTER 3

Antimalarial, Antibiotics, Antibacterial and Antifungal Drugs

Abstract: This chapter deals with the class of aminoquinolines or quinolone antimalarial, antibiotic, antibacterial and antifungal drugs. Brand names of the antimalarial agent (*e.g.* Chloroquin, Primaquine), antifungal agent (*e.g.* Fluconazole), antibiotic agent (Nalidixic acid, Norfloxacin, Chloramphenicol), antibacterial and antifungal agents (Sulphonamides, Sulfamethoxazole, Sulphacetamide, Trimethoprim) along with the uses, mode of action and side effects have been discussed in this chapter. Various synthetic methods have shown for these drug molecules. Different types of name reactions have included as the key for their synthesis.

Keywords: Drug discovery, Pharmaceuticals, Pharmaceutical chemistry, Pharmacology, Pharmacokinetics.

ANTIMALARIAL DRUGS

Chloroquine

Chloroquine, a class of aminoquinolines drug, is an antimalarial drug and is marketed as Aralen. It is used to treat malaria, rheumatoid arthritis, systemic lupus erythematosus, and is used in the systemic therapy of amebic liver abscesses [20a]. It works well for all types of malaria caused by *Plasmodium vivax, Plasmodium ovale* and *Plasmodium malariae*, except disease caused by *Plasmodium falciparum,*[13, 20e], resistant to chloroquine. Chloroquine is taken orally once a day per week, not more or less as that of the prescribed dose on the same day of the week. Overdose of chloroquine may cause headache, drowsiness, nausea, vomiting, vision changes, seizure, slow heart rate, weak pulse, fainting, red or purple skin rash, slow breathing.

Samir Kumar Mandal and Rebeca Ghanta

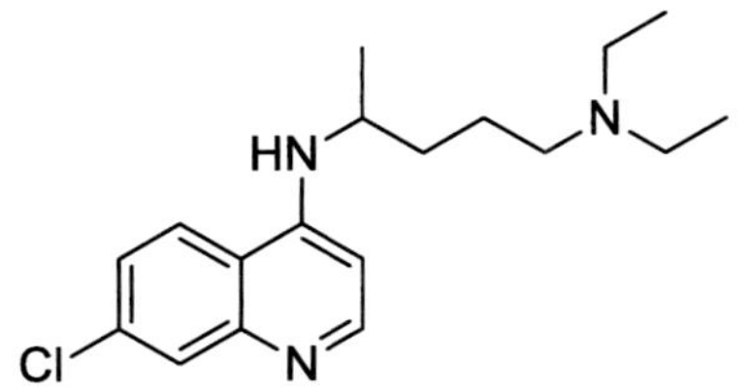

N^4-(7-chloroquinolin-4-yl)-N^1,N^1-diethylpentane-1,4-diamine
(Chloroquine)

It works by interfering with the growth of parasites in the red blood cells of the human body [13]. Chloroquine, being alkaline in nature, inhibits the parasitic enzyme heme polymerase that converts the toxic heme into non-toxic hemozoin. This helps to accumulate toxic heme within the parasite.

Synthesis [20]

Gould–Jacobs Reaction

Gould–Jacobs reaction is well known for the construction of quinolines and 4-hydroxyquinoline derivatives. The Gould-Jacobs reaction begins with the condensation/substitution of the aromatic amine group with alkoxy methylene-malonic ester or acyl malonic ester and produces anilidomethylenemalonic ester. Diester is cyclized to form 4-hydroxy-3-carboalkoxyquinoline. The carboalkoxy group of 4-hydroxy-3-carboalkoxyquinoline is removed on saponification and then decarboxylation gives 4-hydroxyquinoline.

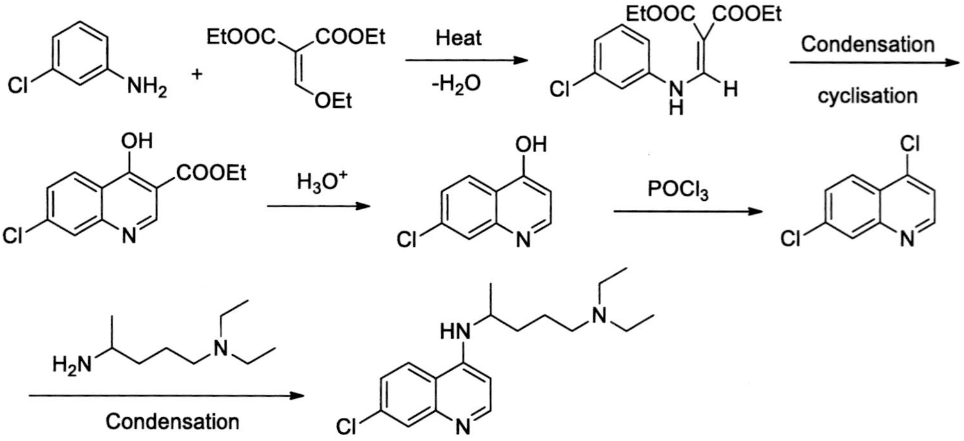

Chloroquine is synthesized from the sequential condensation reaction starting from m-chloroaniline. m-Chloroaniline condenses with formic acid resulting N-aryl formamide. The formyl group further condenses with another molecule of m-chloroaniline to form imine, which is subsequently exchanged with diethyl malonate. The diester undergoes thermal condensation-cyclisation-decarboxylation reaction with the formation of a hydroxyl-quinoline derivative easily. The hydroxy-group is replaced easily with an aminoalkyl group using sequential $POCl_3$ and suitable alkyl amine under aromatic nucleophilic substitution. $POCl_3$ serves here to introduce a better leaving group for the purpose of amine group introduction.

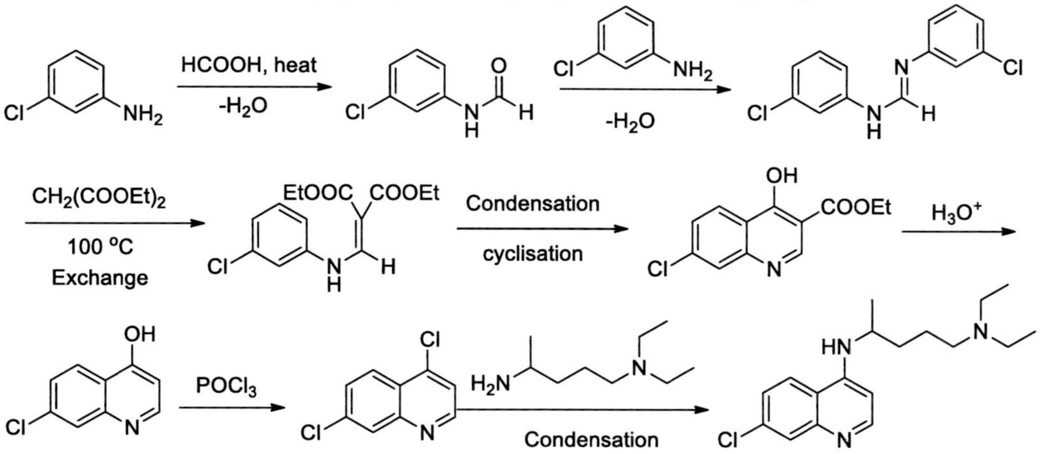

Primaquine

Primaquine [21], a class of aminoquinolines drug, is a medication used to treat malaria and Pneumocystis pneumonia by disrupting plasmodium mitochondria. This is used as a co-drug with chloroquine in treating all cases of malaria. Overdoses of primaquine may cause abdominal pain, hemolytic anemia in G6PD deficiency, nausea, vomiting, rash, dizziness, *etc.* It is absorbed in the body very well and excreted by urine [3, 5].

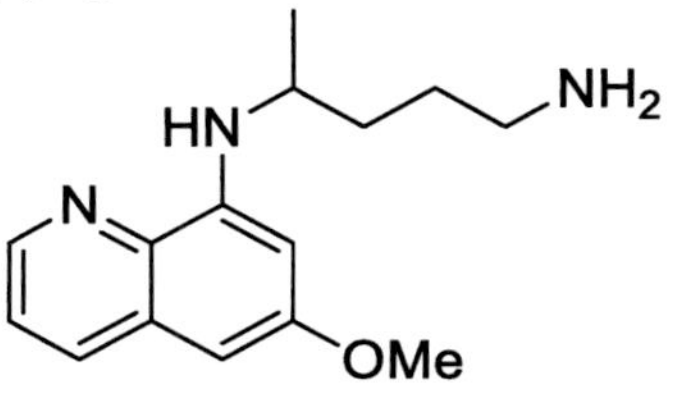

N[4]-(6-methoxyquinolin-8-yl)pentane-1,4-diamine
(Primaquine)

Malaria parasites break down a part of the red blood cells into two parts; haem and globin. Haem is toxic to the malaria parasite. To prevent it from being damaged, the malaria parasite produces a chemical which converts the toxic haem into a non-toxic product [13]. Primaquine interferes with the part of the parasite, which is involved in the production of energy, and consequently, the parasite dies without energy production.

Synthesis

Potassium salt of phthalimide is used as a nucleophile to replace primary alkyl bromide selectively. Secondary bromine is then replaced with an aromatic amine to give an N-alkylated product. Hydrolysis of N-alkylated compound produces primaquine [21].

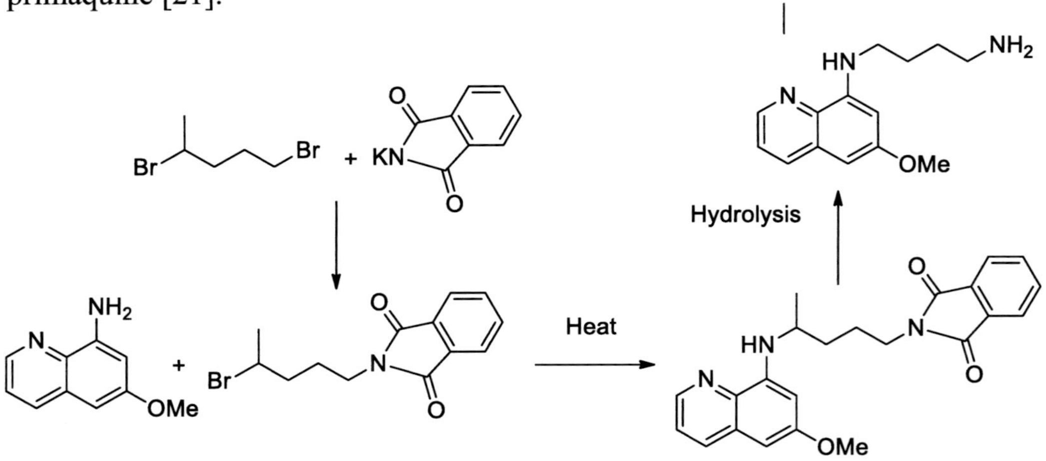

ANTIBIOTICS

Nalidixic Acid

Nalidixic acid, a class of quinolone drug, is the first member of an oral antibacterial agent and is marketed as NegGram® [13, 15]. It was discovered by George Lesher and his coworker during the synthesis of chloroquinone. Since 1962, *Nalidixic acid* has been using for the treatment of urinary tract infections caused by certain bacteria, namely *E. Coli*, *Enterobacter* species, *Klebsiella* species. It is better to not use the medicine if the patients suffer from allergies to medicine or using chemotherapy. Nowadays, this quinolone drug is least often used as more effective agents are available and is more susceptible to bacterial resistance. Overdose of nalidixic acid may cause diarrhea, dizziness, drowsiness, feeling of a whirling motion, headache, nausea, rash, stomach pain or discomfort and vomiting [3, 5].

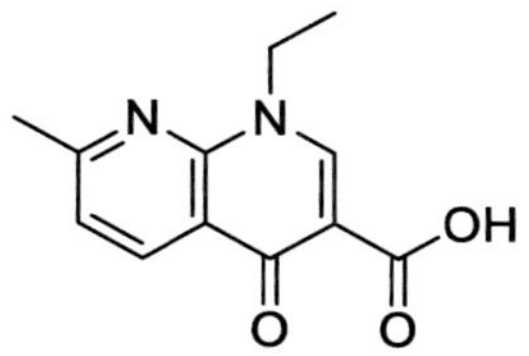

1-ethyl-1,4-dihydro-7-methyl-4-oxo-1,8-naphthyridine-3-carboxylic acid
(Nalidixic acid)

It acts in abacteriostatic manner (inhibits the growth of bacteria or their reproduction) when used in low concentration. In higher concentration, it is bactericidal (kills bacteria instead of inhibiting their growth) in the urinary tract by stopping the production of essential proteins needed for the survival of the bacteria. Its active metabolite, hydroxynalidixic acid, binds strongly, but reversibly to DNA, interfering with the synthesis of RNA and, consequently, with protein synthesis. This antibacterial agent selectively and reversibly blocks DNA replication in susceptible bacteria. In addition to that, nalidixic acid and related antibiotics inhibit a subunit of DNA gyrase and topoisomerase IV.

Norfloxacin

Norfloxacin, a class of 2nd generation fluoroquinolones drugs (others are ofloxacin, ciprofloxacin, lomefloxacin), is an antibiotic drug and is marketed as Noroxin® [15]. It is used for the treatment of different complicated bacterial infections of the prostate or urinary tract, including gonorrhea, by inhibiting bacterial DNA replication as it binds with enzyme DNA gyrase. The experimental result suggests that the fluorine atom at the 6-position increases potency against gram-negative organisms, and the piperazine moiety at the 7-position is responsible for the anti-pseudomonal activity. It is removed through metabolism, biliary excretion, and renal excretion [5, 13, 22].

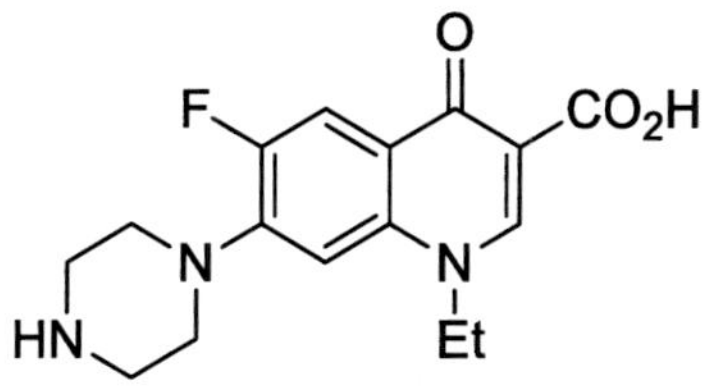

1-ethyl-6-fluoro-4-oxo-7-(piperazin-1-yl)-1,4-dihydroquinoline-3-carboxylic acid
(Norfloxacin)

It inhibits bacterial DNA replication as it binds with the enzyme DNA gyrase. This causes the release of double-stranded DNA break and thereby bacterial cell death

(Fig. **1**). It causes minimum side effects as it is more selective towards bacterial DNA gyrase than for mammalian and has a broader clinical application compared to the non-fluoroquinolone drug [3].

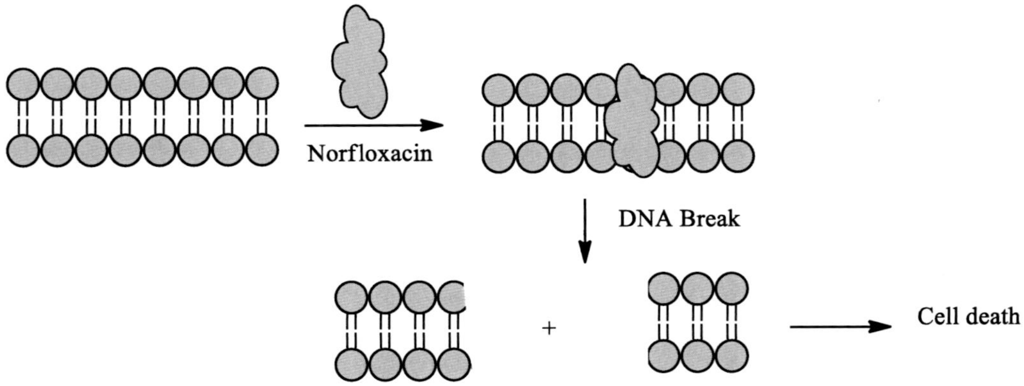

Fig. (1). DNA break and cell death by Norfloxacin.

Synthesis

Norfloxacin is synthesized following Gould–Jacobs reaction protocol [3, 22b]. In this process, saponification is carried out after the N-alkylation of the naphthyridine ring. Nucleophilic substitution of the Cl-group by piperazine gives norfloxacin. This process is being assisted by the F-group.

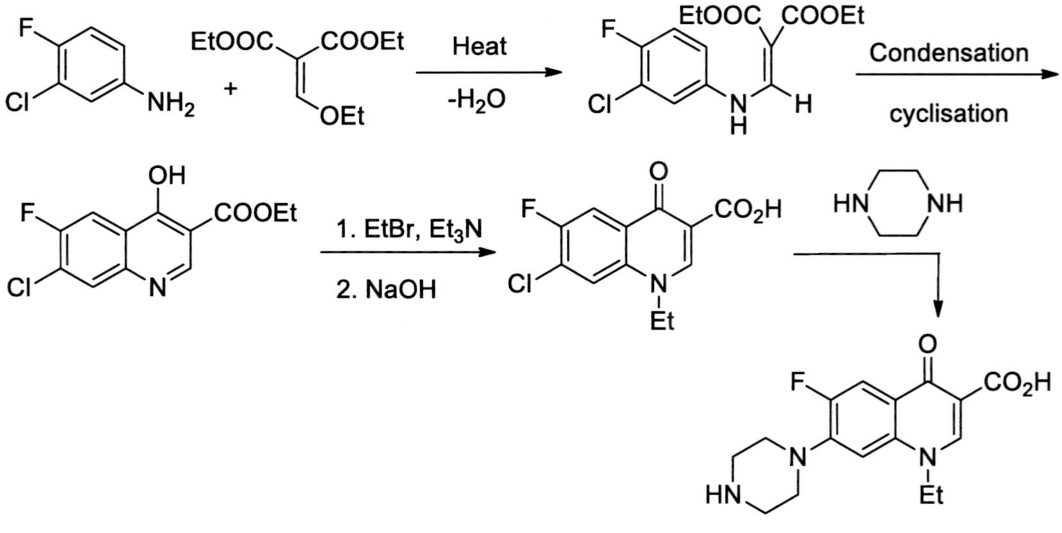

Chloramphenicol

Chloramphenicol is the first broad-spectrum antibiotic (Amphenicol-class Antibacterial) derived by Burkholder and Gottlieb from bacterium *Streptomyces venezuelae* in 1947. This falls in the category of bacteriostatic, which stops the reproduction of bacteria [3, 6, 23d]. This drug is used, under the brand name Chloromycetin®, Econochlor®, Ocu-Chlor®, mainly for the treatment of cholera, meningitis, plague, typhoid fever but also used as eye drops or ointment to treat bacterial conjunctivitis [13, 15]. It causes serious side effects in many cases such as neurotoxicity, hematologic disorders like bone marrow depression and aplastic anemia, nausea, diarrhea, *etc.* Generally, it is not recommended at the end of pregnancy and during breastfeeding. Chloramphenicol should only be used for serious infections in which other medicines do not work. In 2007, WHO listed this as 'probable human carcinogen' based on repeated report to restrict the use.

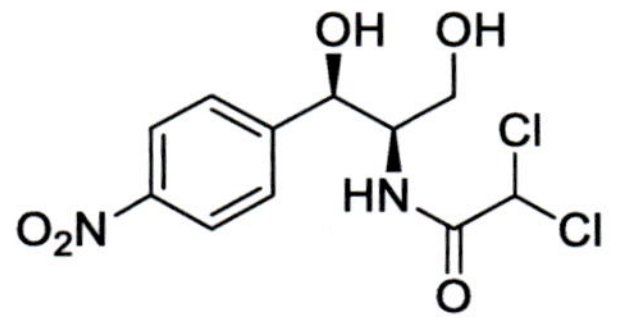

2,2-dichloro-*N*-((1*R*,2*R*)-1,3-dihydroxy-1-(4-nitrophenyl)propan-2-yl)acetamide
(Chloramphenicol)

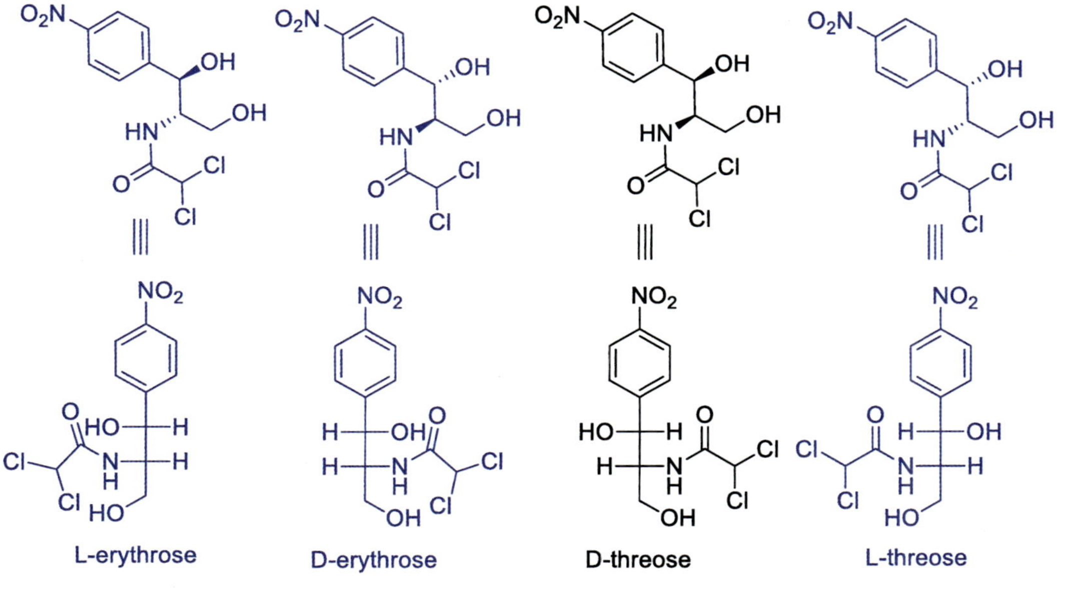

It is regarded as the derivative of 1,3-propane-diol with two substituents, namely, *p*-nitrophenyl (at one extreme carbon) and dichloroacetamide (at middle carbon). Out of four optical isomers with two stereocentres, only the D-threose form is biologically active and naturally available, but the other three are not [4, 5].

It disperses through the bacterial cell wall and reversibly binds to the bacterial ribosomal subunit. This inhibits bacterial protein synthesis by interfering with the activity of peptidyl transferase, a transacylase involved in bacterial peptidoglycan synthesis. As a result, it prevents the transfer of amino acids to the growing peptide chains of bacteria.

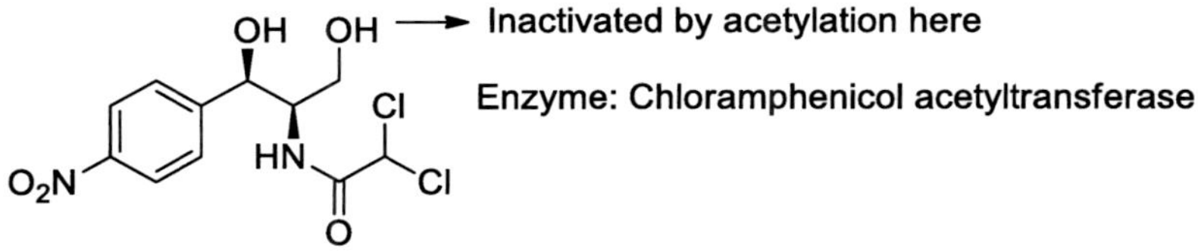

Synthesis

Chloramphenicol is a metabolic product of *Streptomyces venezuelae.* It was extracted from the fermentation broth separated from the mycelium by means of ethyl acetate at the acid reaction. Ethyl acetate is evaporated to dryness and extracted with diethyl ether. The ether solution is then chromatographed using alumina and the ethereal solution obtained as effluent is evaporated. This residue is then extracted with water and agitated with petroleum ether to remove impurities. Crystal of chloramphenicol is obtained when it is concentrated.

But, it is synthesized industrially *via* several methods.

Park Method

Chemically, this is synthesized enantioselectively using the Horner–Wadsworth–Emmons olefination, followed by Sharpless asymmetric dihydroxylation, azide assisted epoxide ring opening and Staudinger reaction as key steps. Amine, produced after the Staudinger reaction, which a very mild reaction for selective reduction of azide, was converted into amide bond in the final step to get chloramphenicol [7, 23a].

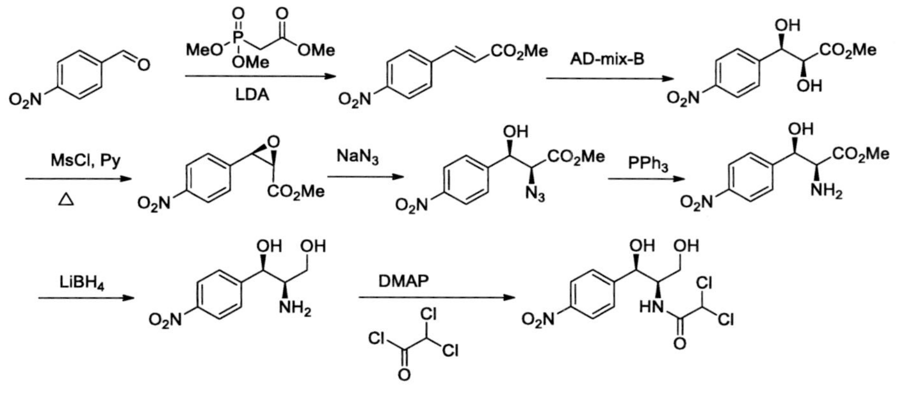

Troutman Method

Troutman Method [23b] is relatively lengthy but one of the easiest routes [10b]. Paranitroacetophenone on alpha–bromination followed by amination with hexamethylenetetramine gives alpha-aminoacetophenone. Then hydroxymethyl group is introduced with formaldehyde, and reduction of the carbonyl group with Raney nickel or *via* the Meerwein–Ponndorf–Verley (MPV) process results in a racemic amino-diol compound. Diastereomeric separation gives (R,R)-amino-diol. Amine is treated with 2,2-dichloroacetyl chloride to get optically pure Chloramphenicol.

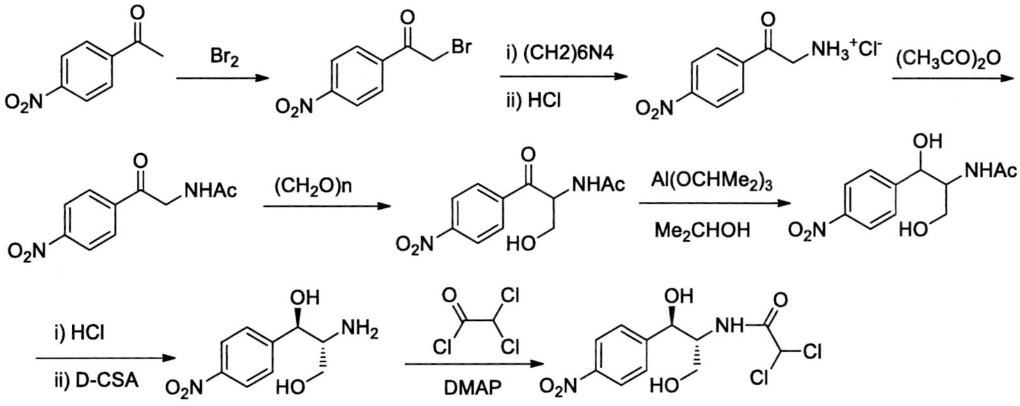

Hoffman-La Roche Method

Hoffman-La Roche described the synthesis starting from ethyl ester of D-threose-β-phenylserine [23c]. The carbonyl group is reduced after blocking the free amine and the hydroxyl group *via* the isoxazole group. Then, the acid hydrolysis results in free amino diol. The amine group is transformed into amide using methyl dichoroacetate. Free 1, 3-diol is again protected by the acetyl group for nitration and then aminolysis results in the desired optically pure chloramphenicol.

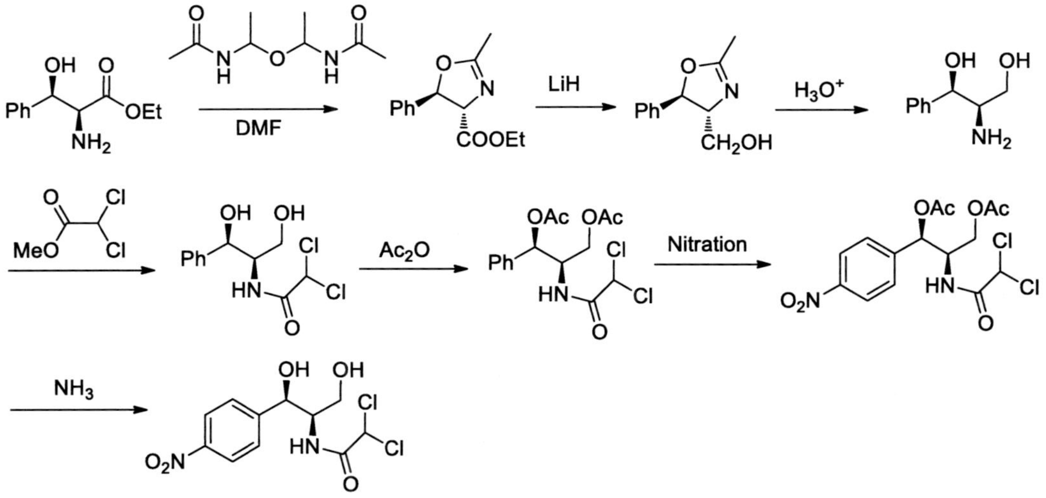

ANTIBACTERIAL AND ANTIFUNGAL DRUGS

Sulphonamides

Sulphonamide is a class of antimicrobial agents with a sulphonamide functional group, formed from the condensation of benzene sulphonic acid and ammonia. These drugs, also known as a sulfa or sulpha drug, are used under the brand name Gantrisin® (acetyl sulfisoxazole), Septra® or Bactrim® (combination of two antibiotics, namely, sulfamethoxazole and trimethoprim), Azulfidine® (sulfa-salazine), Sulfadiazine® (sulfadiazine), *etc.*, as bacteriostatic antibiotics [13-15]. They are also used to treat allergies and cough, antifungal and antimalarial functions. They are used orally and are alkaline in nature [24a].

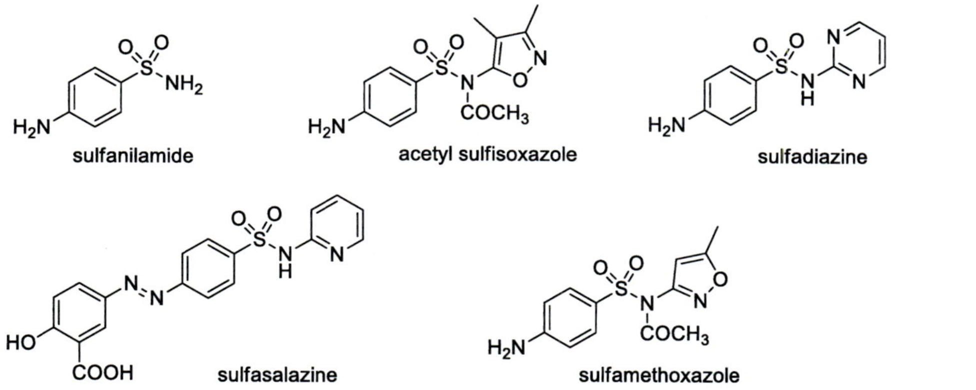

Sulfa drugs

Antibacterial sulfonamides inhibit the bacterial enzyme dihydropteroate synthase (DHPS), which is responsible for folate synthesis. The synthesis of folate is important for the production of anucleic base and, thereby, the synthesis of DNA. Sulphanilamide is very similar in structure to 4-aminobenzenecarboxylic acid (PABA), a precursor of folic acid and is able to inhibit the formation of dihydrofolic acid. Thus, the presence of sulfonamides stops folic acid production and consequently prevents bacterial reproduction. It is selective to bacteria as no folate synthesis in the human body occurs [13, 20e].

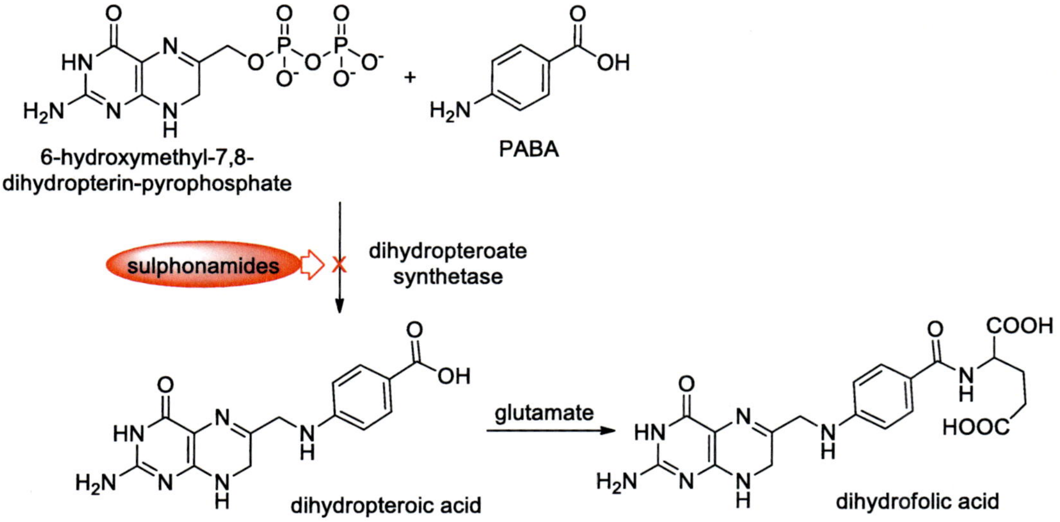

Synthesis

Aniline is initially converted into an acetanilide group for controlling the sulphonation reaction with chloro-sulphonic acid. The common way of synthesis of sulphonamide is the reaction of sulfonyl chlorides with an amine. Pyridine base acts as a proton sponge in this reaction as it absorbs side product, HCl [7].

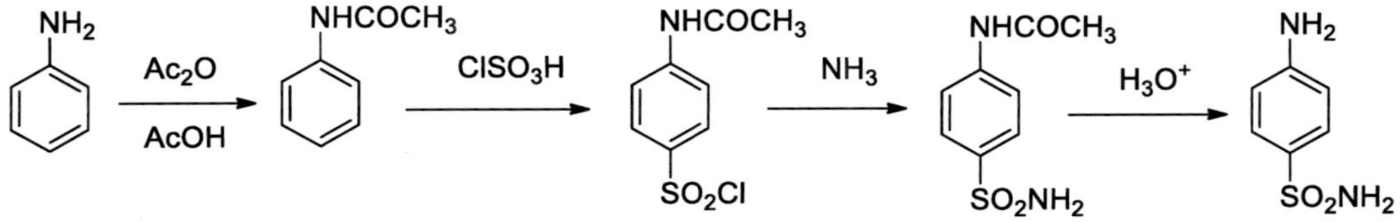

Sulfamethoxazole

Sulfamethoxazole, a sulfonamide, is used as both bacteriostatic and bactericidal for the treatment of bronchitis, prostatitis and urinary tract infections. It contains an isoxazole (1,2-oxazole) unit having a methyl substituent at the 5-position and a 4-aminobenzenesulfonamido group at the 3-position. In most cases, it is used in combination with trimethoprim as a brand name Alcorim-F®, Bactrim®, Ciplin®, Co-Trimoxazole-DS® by showing synergistic action [15]. The most common side effects of the drug are nausea, vomiting, loss of appetite, and skin rashes [7].

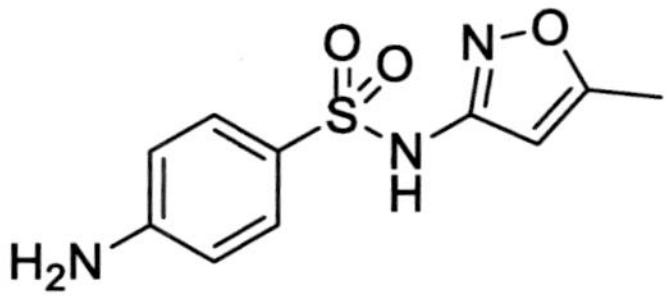

4-amino-*N*-(5-methylisoxazol-3-yl)benzenesulfonamide
(Sulfamethoxazole)

The human body requires folic acid but can't produce the same as they don't have an enzyme like bacteria. Bacterial enzyme dihydropteroate synthase involves in the production of folic acid from *para*-aminobenzoic acid (PABA). Sulfamethoxazole drug competes with *para*-aminobenzoic acid (PABA) for binding to bacterial enzyme dihydropteroate synthase and thus prevents the bacterial synthesis of dihydrofolic acid. This ultimately inhibits bacterial DNA synthesis and destroys the bacteria [3, 5, 13].

Synthesis

Aniline is transformed into acetanilide and then chlorosulphonation results in 4-acetamidobenzene-1-sulfonyl chloride. This acid chloride of sulphanilic acid is treated with 1,2-isoxazole amine (5-methylisoxazol-3-amine) to give acetamido-sulfonamide. Then, in aqueous acid treatment, results in sulfamethoxazole [7].

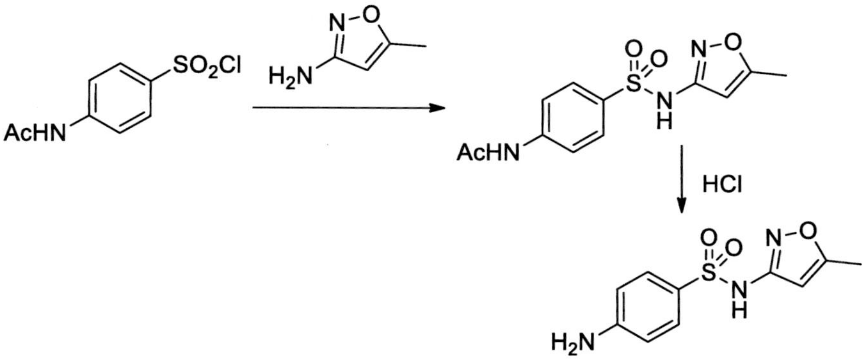

Sulphacetamide

Sulphacetamide, a sulfonamide, is used as bacteriostatic antibiotics for the treatment of acne, seborrheic dermatitis, conjunctivitis (in eye-drop solution) and urinary tract infections.This drug is used under the brand name Bleph®, Ocu-Sulf®, Albucid®, Cetamide®, Klaron® or Ovace® [13, 15]. Application of this drug is restricted during pregnancy, breastfeeding, suffering from herpes. They are used orally and are alkaline in nature. The most common side effects of the drug are irritation, stinging or burning of the skin, nausea, vomiting, dizziness, and headache [5].

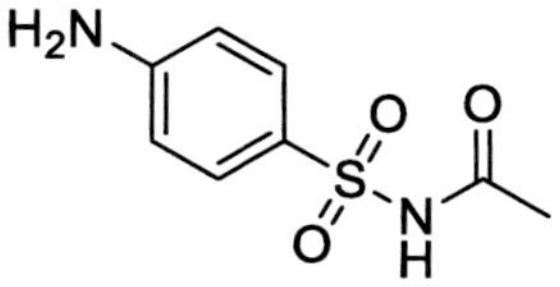

N-(4-aminophenyl)sulfonylacetamide
(Sulfacetamide)

This competes with *para*-aminobenzoic acid (PABA) for binding to bacterial enzyme dihydropteroate synthase and thus prevents the bacterial synthesis of dihydrofolic acid. This ultimately destroys the bacteria [7].

Synthesis

Synthesis of sulphacetamide is achieved either from the reaction of acetamide with 4-aminobenzenesulfonyl chloride or from the reaction of 4-aminobenzenesulfonamide with acetic anhydride.

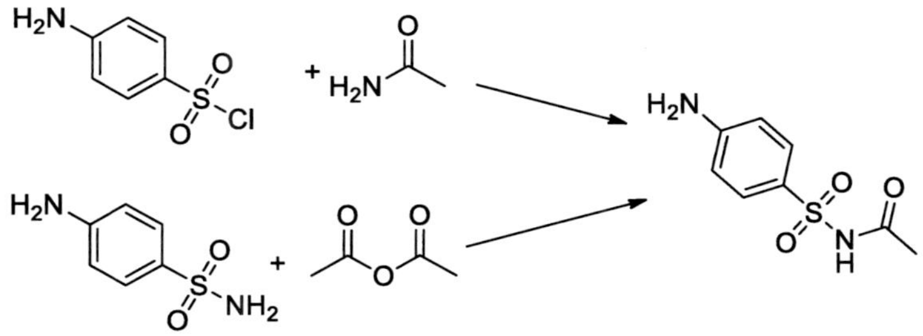

Trimethoprim

Trimethoprim, with pyrimidine core, is an antifungal and antibacterial agent and used as antibiotics for the treatment of urinary tract infections, respiratory tract infections [25a, 3, 5, 7]. This is usually used in combination with sulphonamides to reduce the resistance when used alone. Sometimes it is used singly for the treatment of malaria. This works by killing the bacteria that cause the infection of the urinary tract. It is advised to avoid taking the medicine to patients allergic to trimethoprim, while pregnant and breastfeeding, megaloblastic anemia (caused by folate deficiency). The most common side effects of the drug are itching, mouth sores, muscle weakness, nausea, skin rash, stomach pain, vomiting.

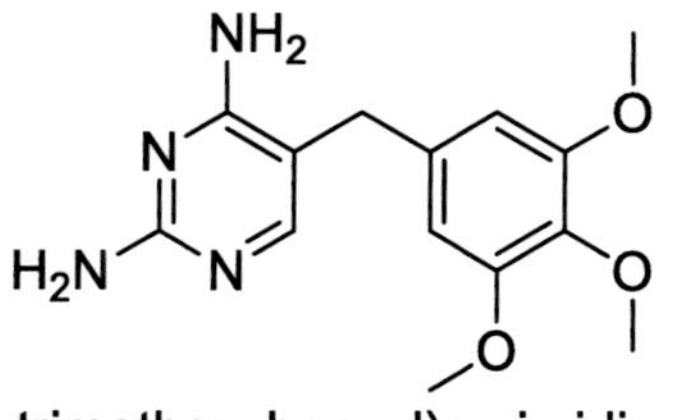

5-(3,4,5-trimethoxybenzyl)pyrimidine-2,4-diamine

(Trimethoprim)

Although both the bacteria and human can reduce dihydrofolic acid (DHF) to tetrahydrofolic acid (THF), the human enzyme is still different. Trimethoprim is a selective pyrimidine inhibitor of bacterial dihydrofolate reductase, it is an antibacterial related to pyrimethamine. Thus trimethoprim interferes with the folic acid metabolism of bacteria by inhibiting dihydrofolic acid (DHF) to tetrahydrofolic acid (THF) and thereby inhibits the growth of bacteria [3, 5, 13].

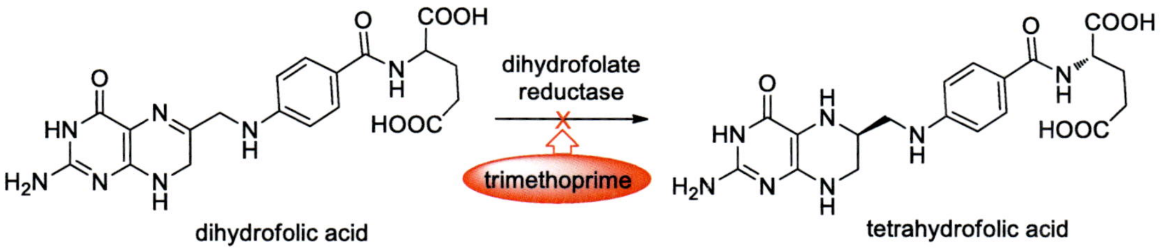

Synthesis

Alkylation of diethylmalonate results in di-ester molecules. One ester group is removed by decarboxylation using NaCl in DMSO (Krapcho decarboxylation). Formylation of ethyl propanoate using ethyl formate and condensation/cyclisation with guanidine gives the pyrimidine containing a hydroxyl group. Conventional amination of pyrimidine gives trimethoprim [7].

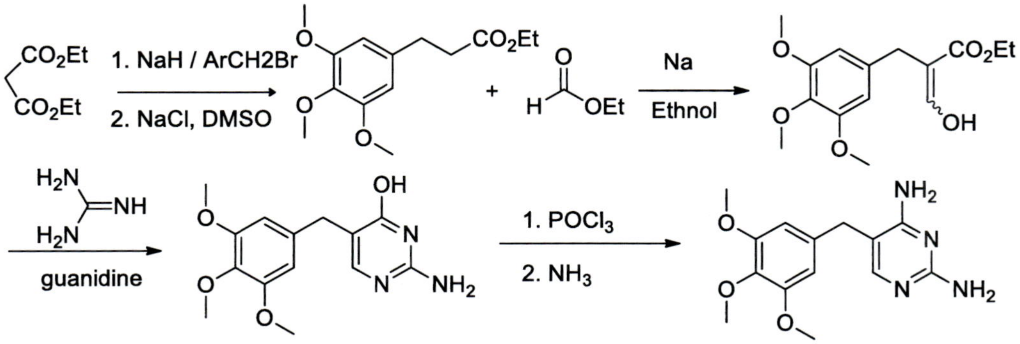

Another method involves condensation of trimethyl benzaldehyde and ethyl cyanoacetate to give 2-cyano propenoate. This on hydrogenation and condensation with guanidine gives hydroxyl pyrimidine. Subsequent amination of pyrimidine gives trimethoprim [25].

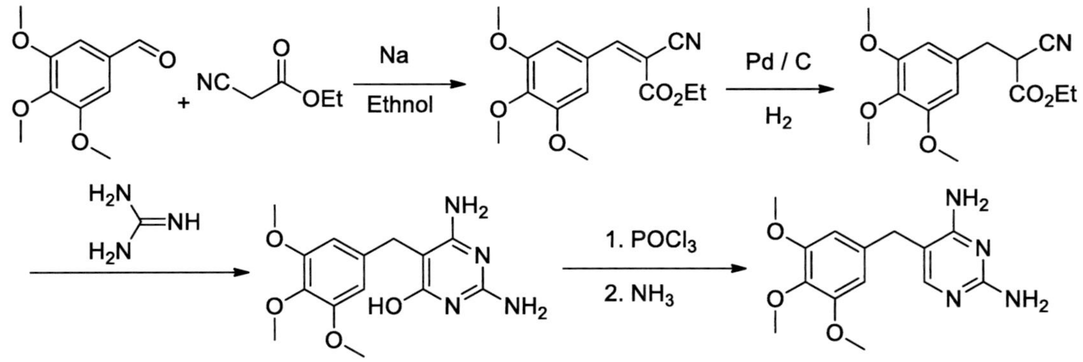

In some cases, arylacrylonitrile is produced from the benzyl alcohol with malononitrile and then condensation with guanidine gives trimethoprim [7].

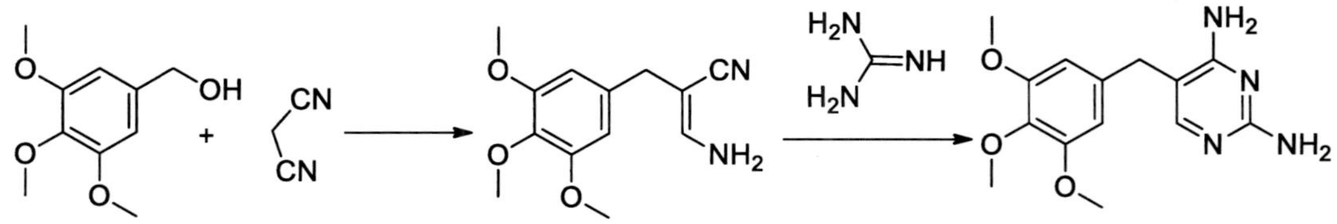

ANTIFUNGAL DRUGS

Fluconazole

Fluconazole, a class of 1,2,4-triazoles, is an example of a modern antifungal drug developed by Pifzer in 1981 [7, 26c-d]. It contains two triazole units and marketed as Diflucan®. It shows fungicidal activity towards several microorganisms like *Candida albicans, Candida glabrata* (Many strains are intermediately susceptible), *Candida parapsilosis, Candida tropicalis* by inhibiting the cell wall synthesis [13, 15]. It is used for the treatment of both systemic and superficial fungal infections in a variety of tissues, including urinary tract infections or vaginal yeast infections [13]. Fluconazole has several advantages (*e.g.*, oral use) over other imidazole- and triazole-class antifungal drugs, including minimum side effects as it is more selective for *fungal* cytochrome P-450 enzymes than for a variety of mammalian cytochrome P-450 enzymes. It forms metabolite minimally, and the majority of intake is removed through renal excretion [5].

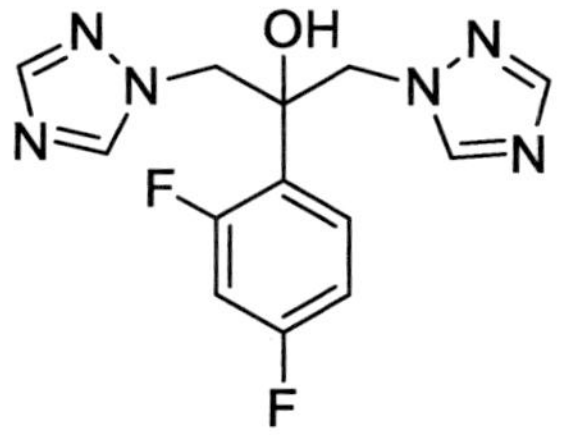

2-(2,4-difluorophenyl)-1,3-di(1*H*-1,2,4-triazol-1-yl)propan-2-ol
(Fluconazole)

Fluconazole selectively inhibits fungal cytochrome P450 dependent enzyme *lanosterol 14-α-demethylase.* This affects the conversion of *lanosterol* to *ergosterol,* necessary for fungal cell wall synthesis. The nitrogen atom of fluconazole binds with the iron atom in the heme group of lanosterol 14-α-demethylase, and consequently, forms an abnormal cell wall of fungi [5, 13].

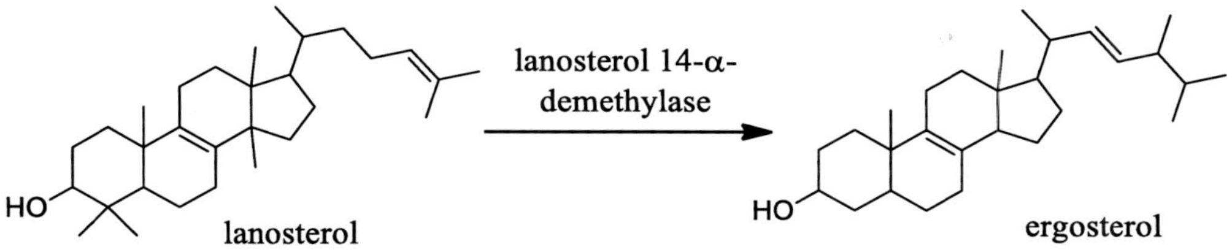

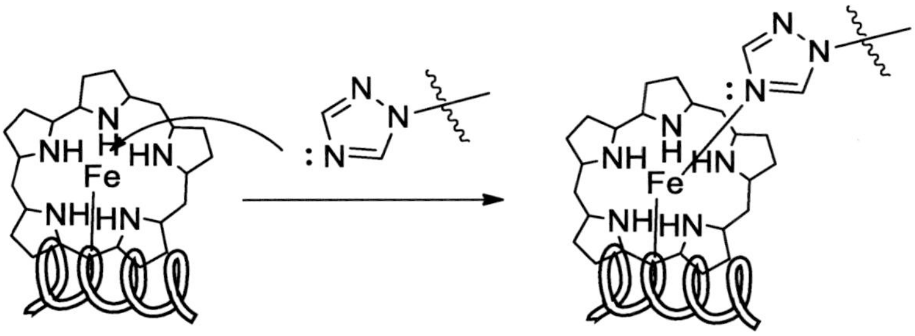

lanosterol 14-α-demethylase lanosterol 14-α-demethylase & fluconazole

Synthesis

It is produced from the fluoro-arene containing α-haloketone. α-Haloketone is prepared from 1,3-difluorobenzene and chloroacetyl chloride under Friedel-Craft reaction. Halide of α-chloroketone is being replaced by one 1,2,4-triazole unit in the presence of a weak base like $NaHCO_3$ or Et_3N. Another 1,2,4-triazole unit is added to the epoxide prepared from the sulfur ylide (Corey-Chaykovsky Reagent). A continuous, two-reactor, three-step synthesis of fluconazole from 2-chloro-2′,4′-

difluoroacetophenone is also in the literature without any intermediate separation or purification [7, 17].

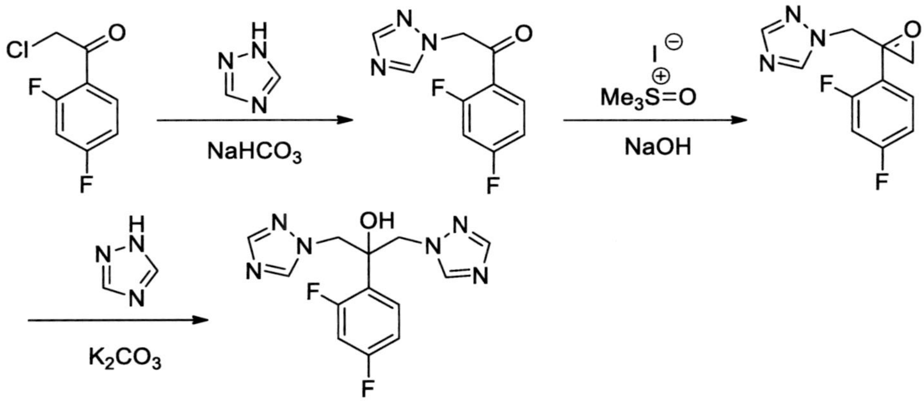

In another way, the 1,3-diester molecule is produced *via* aromatic nucleophilic substitution from diethyl malonate. Difluoro-substitution accelerates the easy removal of iodide in the presence of potassium tertiary butoxide. This diester compound is reduced and tosylated to give the appropriate substrate for further substitution reaction. Consecutive substitution of the *di*-tosylated compound with 1,2,4-trizole gives Fluconazole [26a-b].

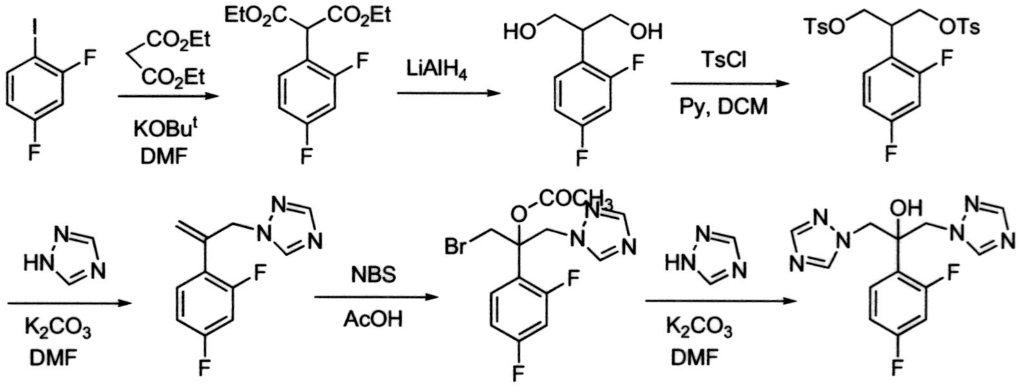

CHAPTER 4

Central Nervous System Drugs, Cardiovascular, Antilaprosy, Antiviral Drugs, HIV-AIDS Related Drugs

Abstract: This chapter deals with the central nervous system (*e.g.* Phenobarbital, Diazepam), cardiovascular (*e.g.* Glyceryl trinitrate), antilaprosy (*e.g.* Dapsone), antiviral (*e.g.* Acyclovir), HIV-AIDS (*e.g.* AZT- Zidovudine) related drugs. Their brand names, brief history of discovery, uses, mode of action and side effects have been discussed to introduce the beginners. In addition, the role of nucleoside analogues *e.g.* Acyclovir, Zidovudine in the chain termination of viral DNA synthesis has been explained in this chapter.

Keywords: Drug discovery, Pharmaceuticals, Pharmaceutical chemistry, Pharmacology, Pharmacokinetics.

CENTRAL NERVOUS SYSTEM DRUGS

Phenobarbital

Earlier convulsive disorders and sedative-hypnotic therapy were based on barbiturates. This is no longer in favor because of their many side effects and their suicide potential. Phenobarbital, due to its increased potency, is used as anti-epileptic drugs discovered in 1912. It is listed in WHO's list of essential medicine that requires for the health system. Phenobarbital is also used to treat trouble sleeping, anxiety, drug withdrawal and control seizures under the brand name Epilan®, Epiphen®, Polytoin-Plus®, *etc.* Controlling and reducing seizures allow performing more normal daily activities, reduce the risk of harm at the time of consciousness, and lessen the life-threatening condition of frequent, repeated seizures. The common side effects are a decreased level of consciousness along with a decreased effort to breathe. It remains effective up to a maximum of 2 days. Phenobarbital usually uses for a short time (no more than 2 weeks) to help calm and sleep. Addiction to a barbiturate drug is very serious and misuse of phenobarbital could be fatal. Phenobarbital is not recommended to a patient having severe liver diseases, severe asthma, a personal or family history of porphyria [3, 5-6].

Samir Kumar Mandal and Rebeca Ghanta

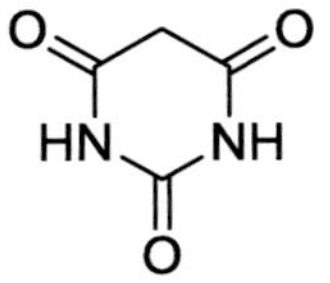

pyrimidine-2,4,6(1*H*,3*H*,5*H*)-trione
(barbiturate)

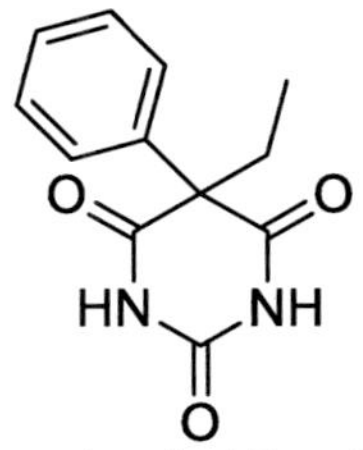

5-ethyl-5-phenylpyrimidine-2,4,6(1*H*,3*H*,5*H*)-trione
(Phenobarbital)

Phenobarbital works by controlling the abnormal electrical activity in the brain at the time of seizure. It depressed the central nervous system by increasing the activity of the inhibitory neurotransmitter, γ-Aminobutyric acid (GABA). It increases the flux of chloride ions into the neuron, which decreases the excitability of the post-synaptic neuron [13].

Synthesis

The most common way of phenobarbital synthesis is base catalysed condensation reactions between a derivative of diethyl malonate and urea [27a]. Benzyl cyanide is converted to phenyl acetic acid ethyl ester by Pinner reaction. Cross Claisen condensation of phenyl acetic acid ethyl ester with diethyl oxalate gives diethyl ester of phenyloxobutandioic acid. This compound is heated to result in diethyl phenylmalonate, which subsequently on alkylation gives phenylethylmalonic diethyl ester. Phenylethylmalonic diethyl ester is condensed with urea in the medium of sodium ethoxide to produce phenobarbital. Condensation of urea with the α-phenyl-α-ethylcyanoacetic ester is also useful for the synthesis of phenobarbital. α-phenyl-α-ethylcyanoacetic ester is easily achieved from the reaction of benzyl cyanide with diethyl carbonate in the presence of a strong base followed by alkylation with ethyl bromide.

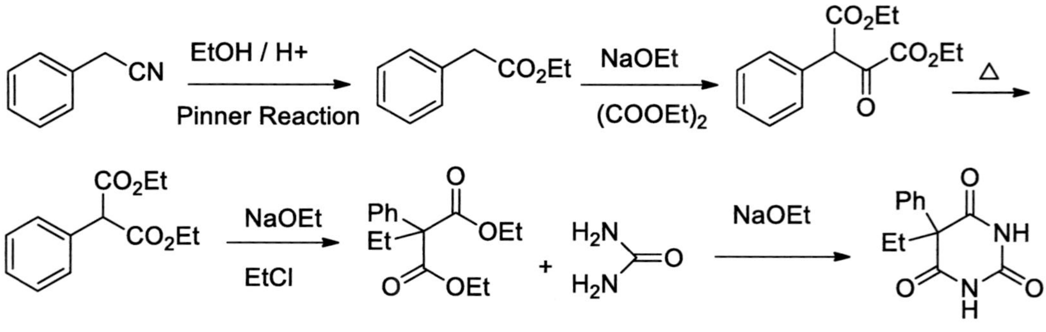

In another way, malonate is alkylated twice in the basic medium. Firstly, malonate is alkylated with ethyl chloride, and secondly, it is alkylated with phenyl chloride. The ethylphenylmalonate is then condensed with guanidine to form animino-barbiturate derivative, which on hydrolysis, yielded phenobarbital [27a, c].

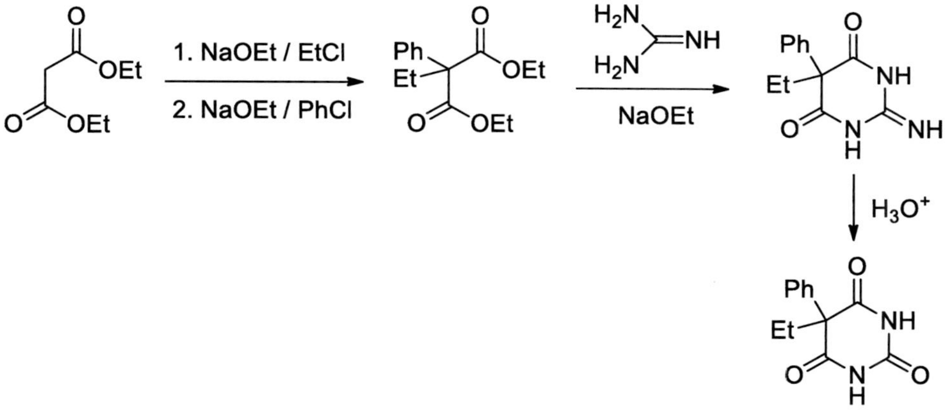

Diazepam

Diazepam, of the benzodiazepine family, was used in 1963 to treat different conditions, *e.g.*, anxiety, alcohol withdrawal syndrome, sedative, muscle spasms, seizures, trouble sleeping, and restless legs syndrome under the brand name Diazepam Intensol®, Valium®, Diastat Acudial®, Diastat®, Alzolam®, Zolax®, *etc* [13, 14]. It is also used for memory loss and keeps the patient in calm status with a long duration of action and provides relief from panic attacks by relaxing the nerves. It shows side effects, *e.g.*, diarrhea, rash, sleepiness and trouble with coordination, decreased breathing, and an increased risk of seizures. Diazepam should not be used during pregnancy and breastfeeding since it may cause fetal abnormalities [3, 5].

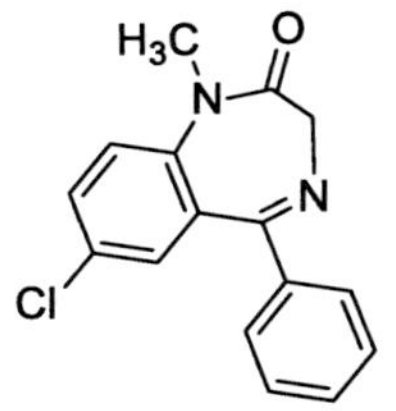

7-chloro-1-methyl-5-phenyl-1*H*-benzo[*e*][1,4]diazepin-2(3*H*)-one
(Diazepam)

Excessive activity in the brain may lead to anxiety or other psychiatric disorders. Gamma-aminobutyric acid (GABA) inhibits activity in the brain. Diazepam works by opening an integral chloride channel, which enhances the effects of GABA in the brain. As a result, anxiety disorder slows down [13, 28b].

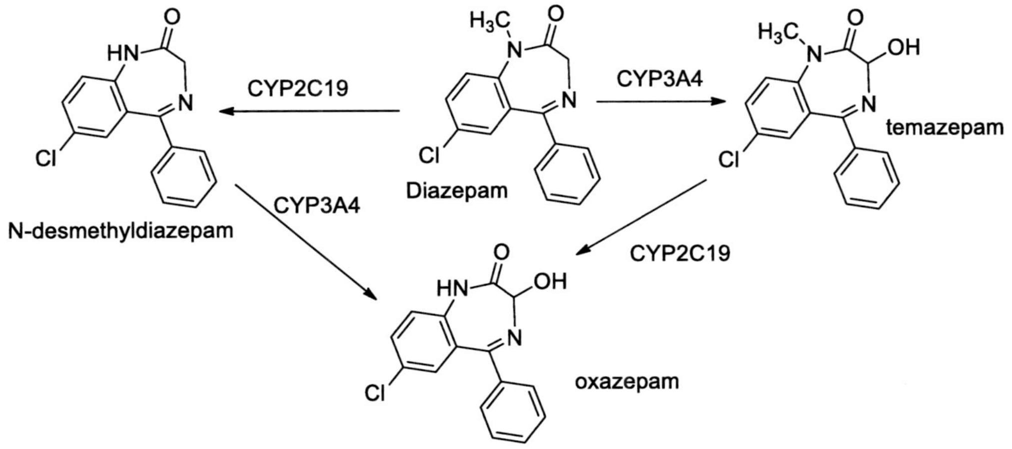

Diazepam on the metabolic process is successively hydroxylated and/or N-demethylated to the active metabolite into temazepam and into N-desmethyldiazepam by CYP3A4 and CYP2C19 enzymes, respectively. Both metabolites are further metabolized to oxazepam. Poor metabolizers of diazepam showed significantly lower clearance than extensive metabolizers after a single oral dose, this causes its long term effect. Diazepam is mainly excreted from the body *via* urine [5].

Synthesis [15]

For the synthesis of benzodiazepine, 5-chloro-isatoic anhydride in dimethylformamide is treated with methyl iodide and produces N-methyl-5-chloro-isatoic anhydride, which on further treatment with glycine and triethyl amine gives cyclic diamide derivative. Acetylation of free amine converts to acetylated compound and then reacts with the Grignard reagent to produce the benzophenone derivative. Benzophenone is converted into oxime followed by refluxing with $NaHSO_3$, and treatment with HCl gives diazepam.

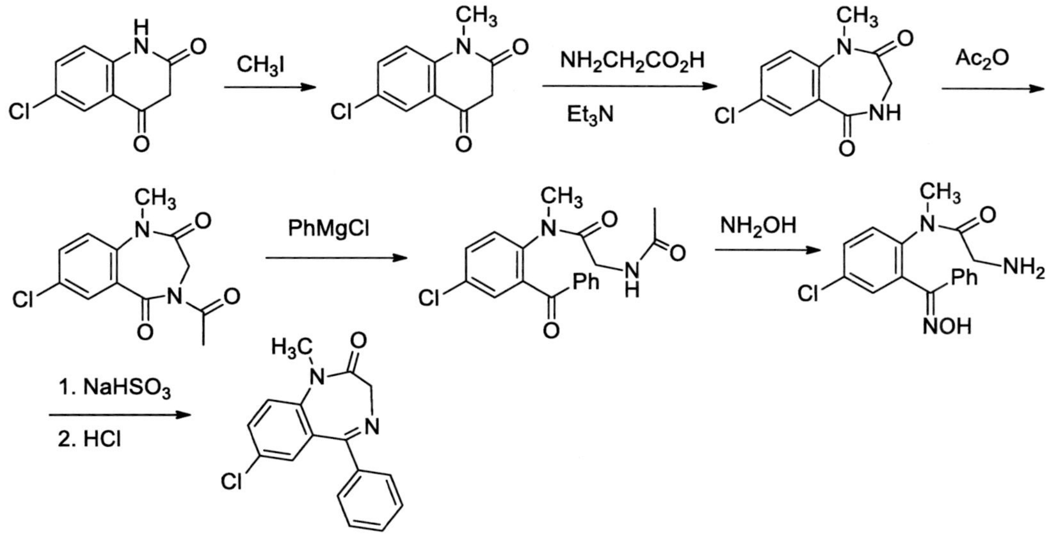

A very simple method where 2-amino-5-chlorobenzophenone is first treated with chloroacetyl chloride and methylation of the free N-H group results in diazepam.

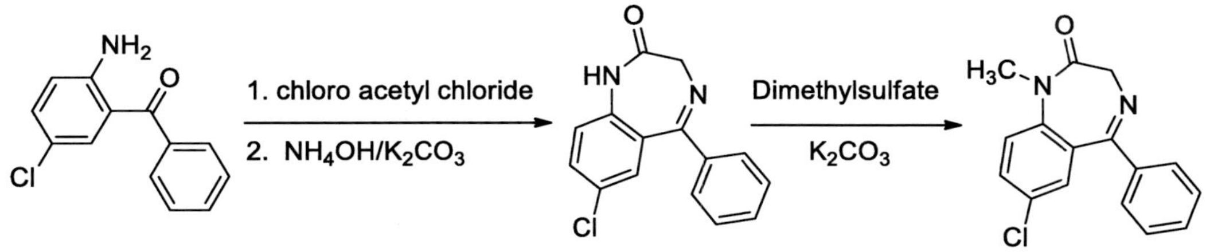

There is some other method related to this where ethyl glycinate is used instead of chloroacetyl chloride. Cyclization of 2-amino-5-chloro-benzophenone with ethyl glycinate in refluxing pyridine followed by methylation results in diazepam. The methylation step is minimized using 2-methylamino-5-chloro-benzophenone as the starting material. The same is achievable by cyclization of 2-methylamino-5-chloro-benzophenone with 2,5-oxazolidinedione, masked glycinate, in methylene chloride [17].

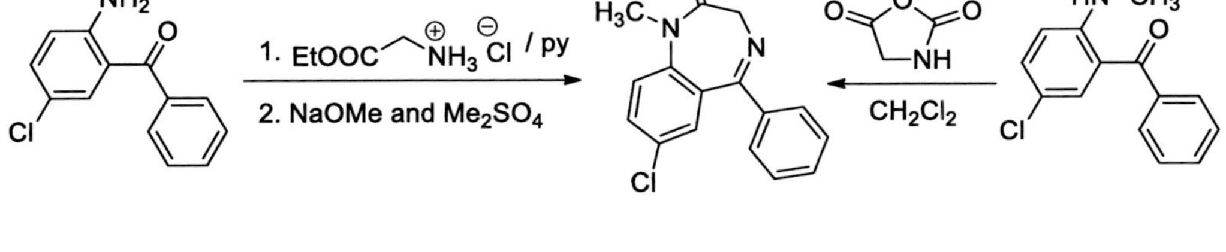

1, 3-dipolar cycloaddition of benzyl cyanide with the 4-nitrochlorobenzene gives the phenyl-benzoisoxazole derivative. Reduction of isoxazole followed by methylation gives benzophenone derivative. Free secondary amine is protected with chloroacetyl chloride and subsequent intramolecular condensation results in diazepam [4b].

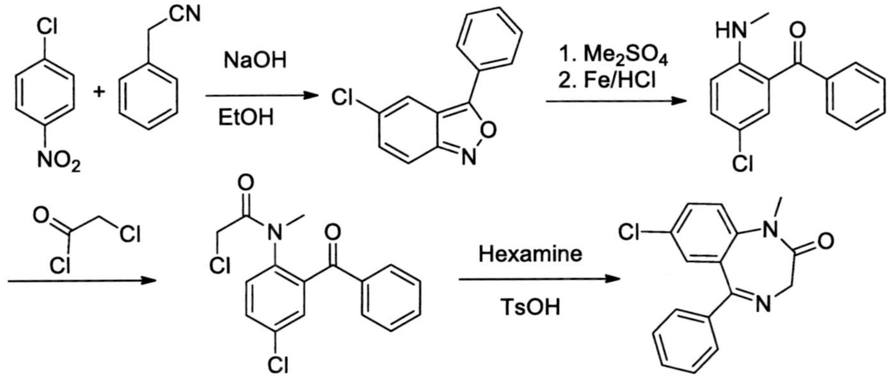

Diazepam has been synthesized from 3-phenyl-5-chloroindole-2-carbonitrile. This process involves methylation-reduction-oxidation-cyclisation. A similar process is useful for the synthesis of diazepam from 3-phenyl-5-chloroindole-2-carboxamide [17].

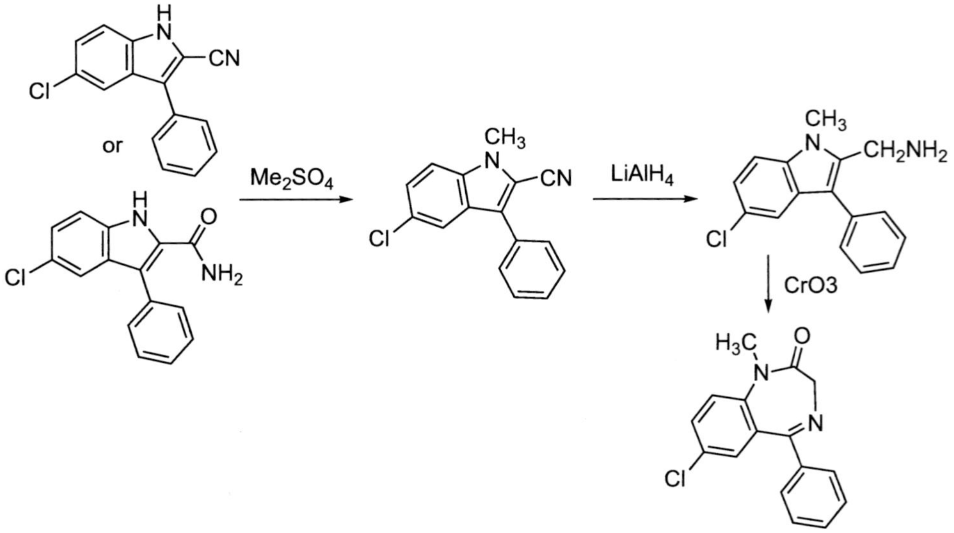

Synthesis of 3-phenyl-5-chloroindole-2-carboxamide is achieved from the condensation of benzyl chloride and ethyl acetoacetate (EAA) in refluxing ethanol followed by cyclization reaction with 4-chloroaniline in HCl. Ethyl 3-phenyl-5-

chloroindole-2-carboxylate could also be prepared from the intramolecular McMurry reaction [17].

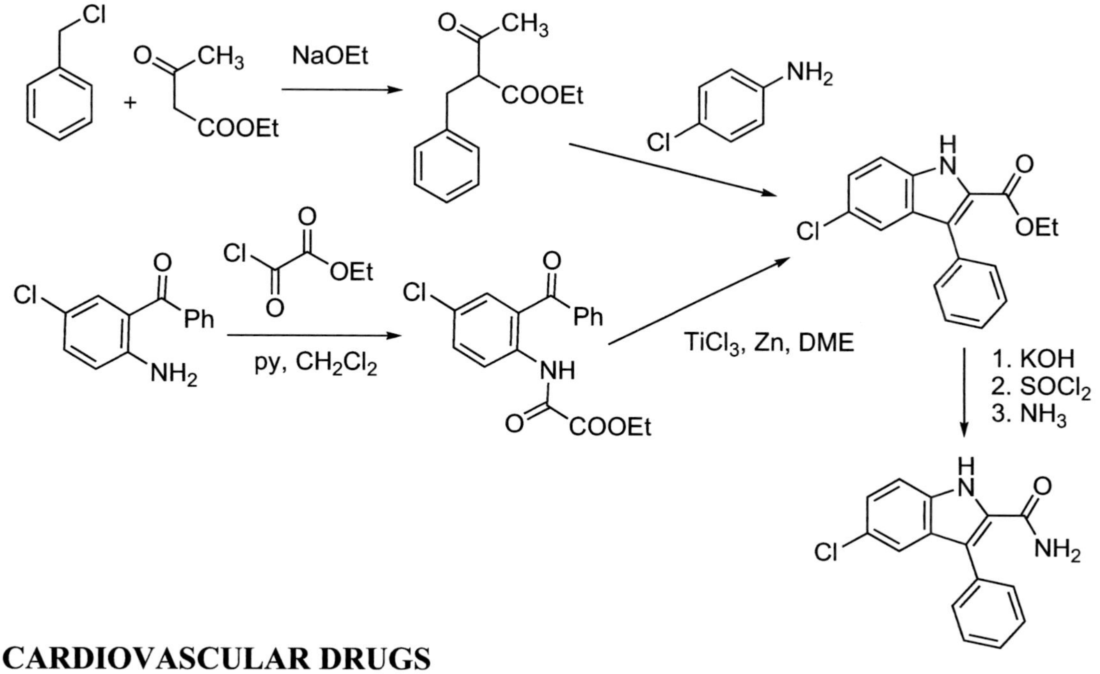

CARDIOVASCULAR DRUGS

Glyceryl Trinitrate

Glyceryl trinitrate (GTN) (considered as organic nitrate), Nitroglycerin (conventional name), was used in 1878 for heart failure, high blood pressure though approved in 2000 to treat and prevent chest pain (angina). It is also used in an ointment to treat the pain that accompanies anal fissures. Glyceryl trinitrate is used in different forms viz. patches, sublingual tablets, sprays and injections under the brand name Angised®, Glynit®, Angispan-TR®, Myovin®, Nitrowok®, Nitroject®, *etc* [3, 5, 13, 15, 29].

Normally, it requires taking medicine every 12h. It is not recommended during pregnancy and breastfeeding. Use of this medicine is also avoided with the symptoms of allergy, anemia, glaucoma, obstructive heart disease, head trauma, intracranial pressure and also patient using the medicine for erectile dysfunction. It causes several side effects, *e.g.*, difficulty in breathing, dizziness and fainting, swelling of the eyes, ears, and inside of nose, severe nausea and vomiting, headache, coma, seizures, change in heart rate, excessive sweating, flushing, severe chest pain, and blurred vision, pale and clammy skin.

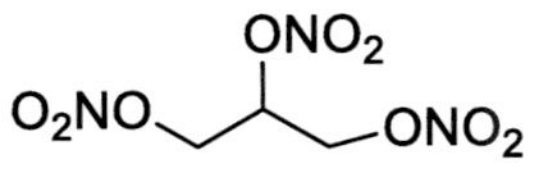

propane-1,2,3-triyl trinitrate
(Glyceryl trinitrate)

It is a prodrug and produces active drug nitric oxide (NO) in the body. A recent study reveals that mitochondrial aldehyde dehydrogenase (ALDH2 or mtALDH) catalyses GTN to produce 1,2-glyceryl dinitrate (GDN) and nitrite (NO_2^-). This subsequently generates NO and/or S-nitrosothiol. However, the degradation route produces 1,3-glyceryl dinitrate (GDN). Production of NO from GTN activates the guanylyl cyclase (GC) and this increases the level of cyclic guanosine monophosphate (cGMP) within the cell. An increased level of cGMP stimulates dephosphorylation of myosin. This initiates the relaxation of smooth muscle cells and causes the coronary artery (blood vessels surrounding the heart) to dilate, increasing blood flow and thereby improving the oxygen supply to the heart. This ultimately leads to a decrease in blood pressure and subsides the chest pain [5, 13, 29].

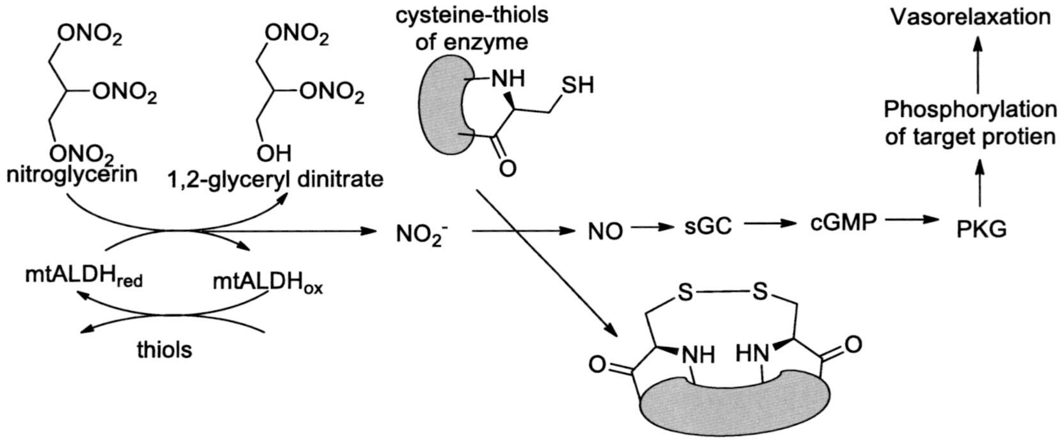

Synthesis

Historically nitroglycerin was first made by Italian chemist Ascanio Sobrero in 1847 by adding glycerin in a mixture of nitric acid and sulfuric acid. This experiment made his face badly scarred due to an explosion. This explosive nature of nitroglycerin was commercialized as dynamite by Swedish scientist Alfred Nobel and became famous when the compound was combined with silica to make it a controlled explosive. Instead of sulphuric acid, phosphoric pentoxide is also useful for the process.

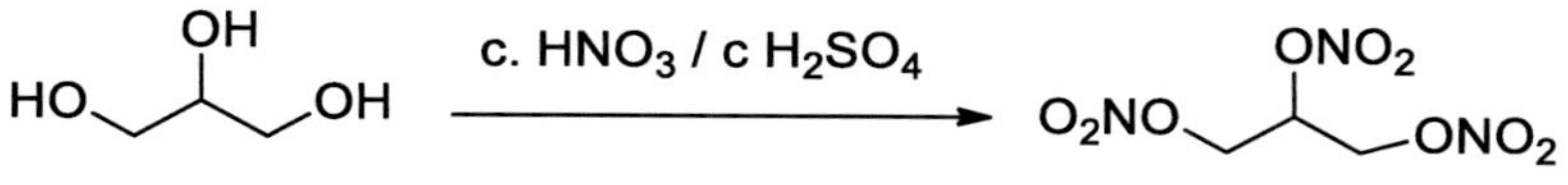

Other Use

(a) ***As dynamite***: Nitroglycerin is commercialized as safer explosive "dynamite" when the compound was combined with silica. Dynamite is an explosive stick that features a wick (a piece of cord that transmits liquid by capillary action) and a blasting cap. The wick is lit (a cause to start burning), which directs to a small explosion when it reaches the blasting cap. When the blasting cap explodes, the nitroglycerin then causes a much larger explosion. The three nitrate groups, powerful oxidizing agents, are bound directly to a hydrocarbon fragment and release a large amount of energy. This exothermic reaction is due to the formation of new strong, stable (multiple bonds) molecules such as N_2 and CO.

(b) **As detonation**: Nitroglycerin having detonation properties, instantaneous destruction of all the molecules in the sample with the rapid expansion of hot gases causes a violent and propagation of destructive explosion, and without solid forms of carbon (soot or smoke), makes it advantageous than other explosives like trinitrotoluene (TNT), which causes. So, it can be used to create 'smokeless powders', which make it advantageous to the armed forces without visionless clouds of billowing smoke and/or smog during a battle [29].

ANTILAPROSY DRUGS

Dapsone

Dapsone is a class of sulfone used to treat Hanson's Disease (leprosy, infectious disease of skin disorder and nerve damage) under the brand name Acnesone Gel®, Dapsone [3, 5, 7, 13]. This is approved by the FDA in 1955 and listed in WHO's list.Leprosy (caused by *Mycobacterium leprae*) remained a burden before the discovery of antibacterial sulfones. Though sulfones and sulfonamides are well known antibacterial agents, dapsone is not very effective for antibacterial activity, but it shows anti-inflammatory, immunosuppressive properties. Both dapsone and sulfones are useful for abroad range of dermatologic and systemic disorders [30c, 14]. Dapsone shows bactericidal as well as bacteriostatic activity to *Mycobacterium leprae*. It requires taking the drug everyday for up to 3 years or for life, otherwise on stopping the medicine, symptoms may return. As an anti-infective agent, it is also useful for the treatment of malaria. The common side effects caused by the drug are unusual behavior, weight gain, loss of appetite, severe allergic reaction, unusual staining, bloody stools, sore throat, nausea, vomiting, skinrash, blurred vision, fever, *etc.* Dapsone should not be used during breastfeeding to prevent the harmful effect of the nursing baby.

Due to less water solubility, it is reacted with bromoacetic acid to give acedisulfone, a water-soluble form. Acedapsone, a prodrug, acetylated form of dapsone, is found to be more effective as it shows both antileprotic and antimalarial activity. Another water-soluble prodrug is its bisulfate adduct made from the formaldehyde bisulifte [7].

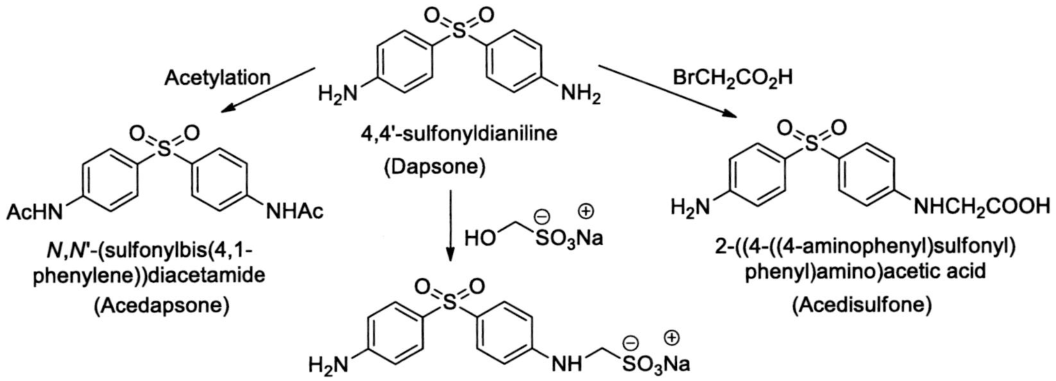

Bacterial enzyme dihydropteroate synthase involves in the production of folic acid from *para*-aminobenzoic acid (PABA). Similar to sulfonamides, dapsone competes with *para*-aminobenzoic acid (PABA) for binding to bacterial enzyme dihydropteroate synthase and thus prevents the bacterial synthesis of dihydrofolic acid. This ultimately inhibits bacterial DNA synthesis and stopping the growth of bacteria [13].

Dapsone is effective in abnormal neutrophil accumulation by interfering with neutrophil chemotactic migration. Systemic dapsone reduces leukotriene B4 and prostaglandins and thereby blocks their inflammatory effects.

Dapsone or diaminodiphenyl sulfone (DDS) is metabolized in the liver *via* acetylation or N-hydroxylation. Cytochrome P-450 (CYP) enzymes yield potentially toxic metabolite hydroxylamine (DDS-NHOH) by N-hydroxylation and N-acetyltransferase (NAT) yields the non-toxic metabolites monoacetyl dapsone (MA-DDS) and diacetyl dapsone by acetylation. Several reports suggest that patients with adverse effects show slow acetylation and fast hydroxylation [5].

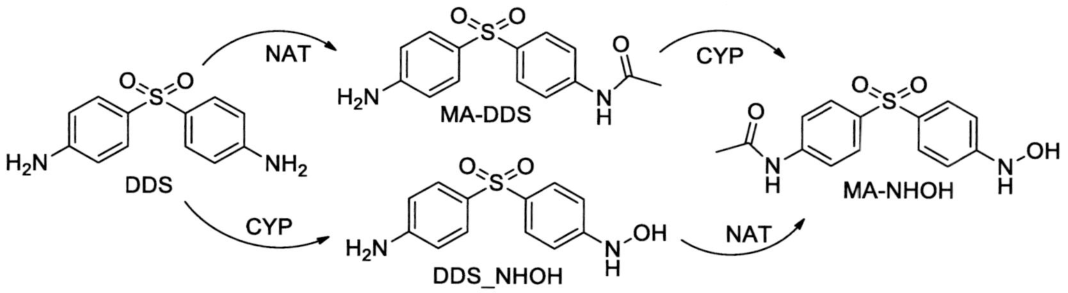

Most of the dapsone and its derivative undergo conjugation with glucuronic acid and then excreted *via* urine [5].

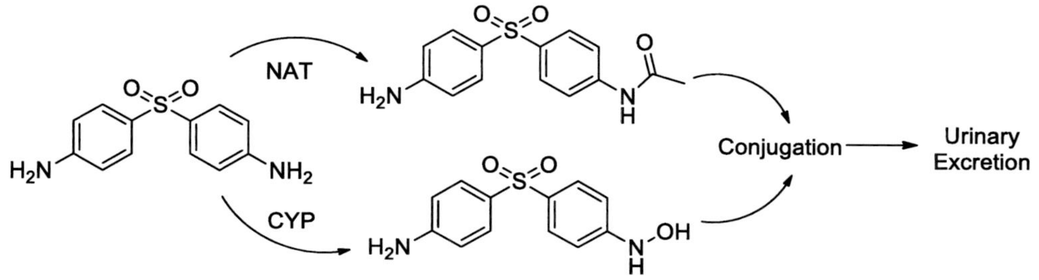

Synthesis

4-chloronitrobenzene is converted into sulfane. Sulfane prepared from 4-chloro-nitrobenzene is oxidized first and then reduced to get 4, 4'-sulfonyldianiline [30c]. The reverse sequence of the process gives unwanted by-product, in some cases, polymeric compound, but acetylation of the amine group followed by oxidation-deacetylation is effective.

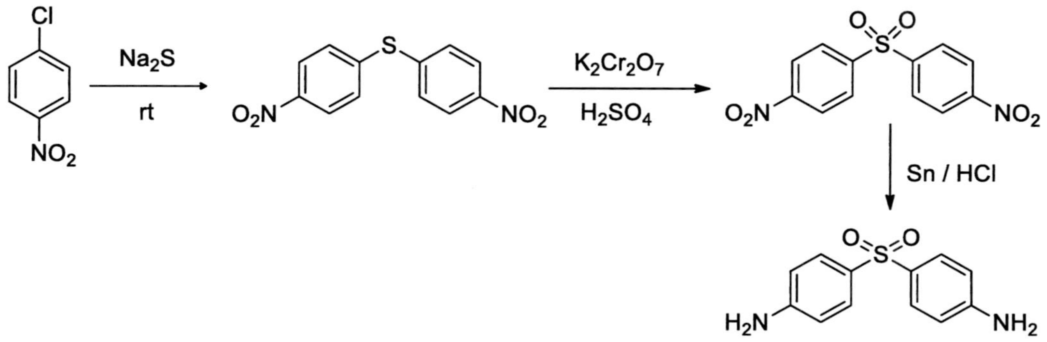

Benzene is condensed with sulfuric acid to result in sulfonyldibenzene. Sulfonyldibenzene is then nitrated using mixed acid followed by reduction giving 4, 4'-sulfonyldianiline.

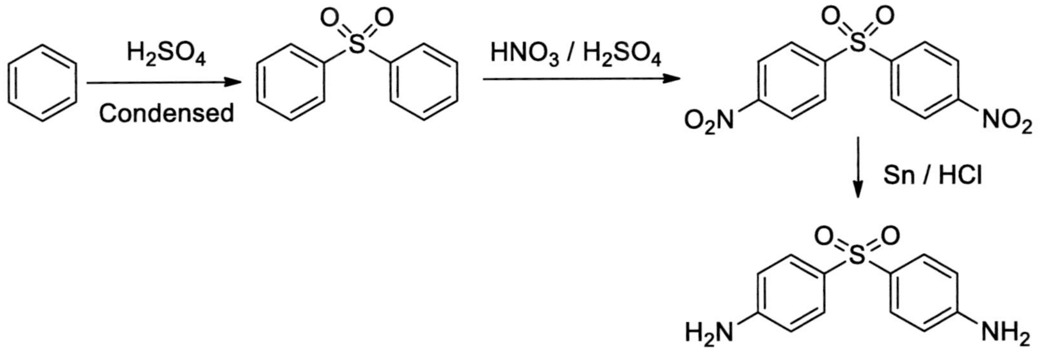

Sodium 4-acetamidobenzenesulfinate is reacted with 4-chloronitrobenzene under SNAr condition at high temperature. Then reduction using tin and hydrochloric acid followed by hydrolysis results in 4, 4'-sulfonyldianiline [30a].

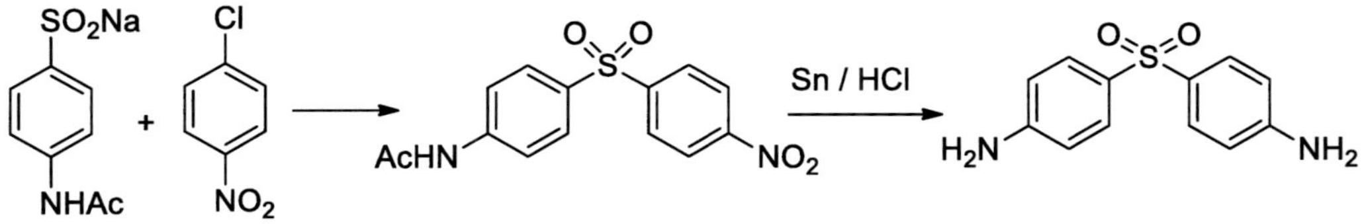

ANTIVIRAL DRUGS

Acyclovir

Acyclovir (Zovirax) is an analogue of the nucleoside guanosine (purine nucleoside) and used as an antiviral agent under the brand name Valtrex® (valacyclovir hydrochloride) [7, 13-15]. It is used to treat infections caused by certain types of viruses such as cold sores around the mouth (caused by herpes simplex), shingles (caused by herpes zoster), and chickenpox (caused by the varicella-zoster virus). It is not used to cure these infections but decreases the severity and length of these outbreaks. Treatment of the viral disease is difficult as viruses use the host cellular mechanism to replicate. Thus, a Nucleoside analogue drug that stops the replication of viral DNA is important for the treatment of viral infection. It decreases the risk of the virus spreading by decreasing the production of the virus's DNA to other parts of the body and thus saves from serious infections [13]. The medicine requires taking it in certain intervals strictly since it works best when the amount of drug in your body is kept at a constant level. The common side effects caused by the drugs are nausea and diarrhea, including serious effects such as kidney problems and low platelet. Overdose may include agitation, coma, seizures, lethargy, and precipitation in renal tubules [5].

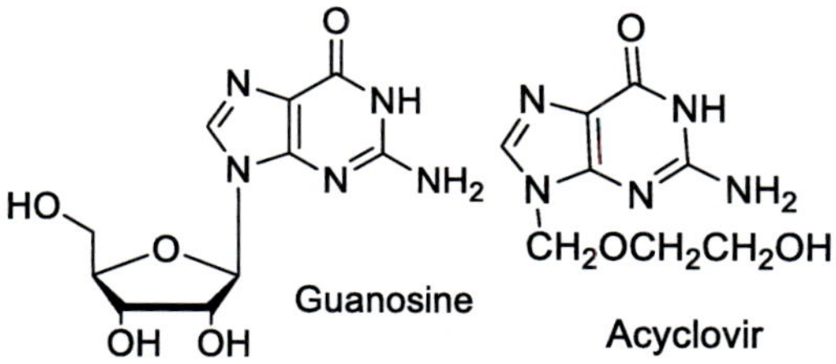

Valacyclovir hydrochloride is administered into the body, which subsequently hydrolysed into active drug acyclovir. Acyclovir works by inhibiting the action of viral DNA polymerase and DNA replication of different herpes virus. It is converted into acyclovir monophosphate by the action of viral thymidine kinase then to the diphosphate form by guanylate kinase. Consequently, acyclovir triphosphate is produced by nucleoside diphosphate kinase, pyruvate kinase, creatine kinase, phosphoglycerate kinase, succinyl-CoA synthetase, phosphoeno-lpyruvate carboxykinase and adenylosuccinate synthetase. Acyclovir triphosphate has a higher affinity for viral DNA polymerase than cellular DNA polymerase and includes into the DNA where the missing 2' and 3' carbons cause chain termination in the synthesis of viral DNA [3, 13].

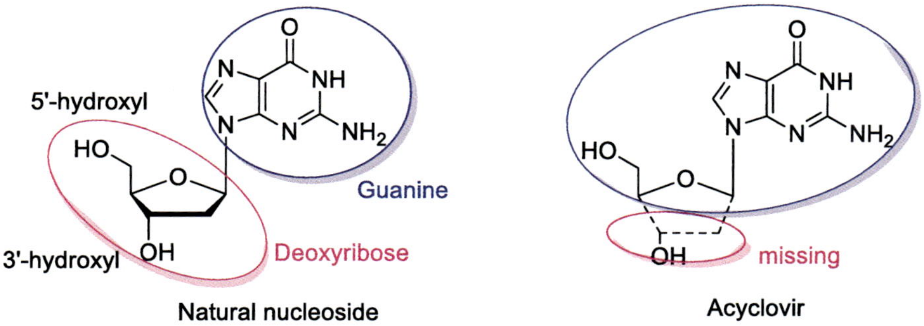

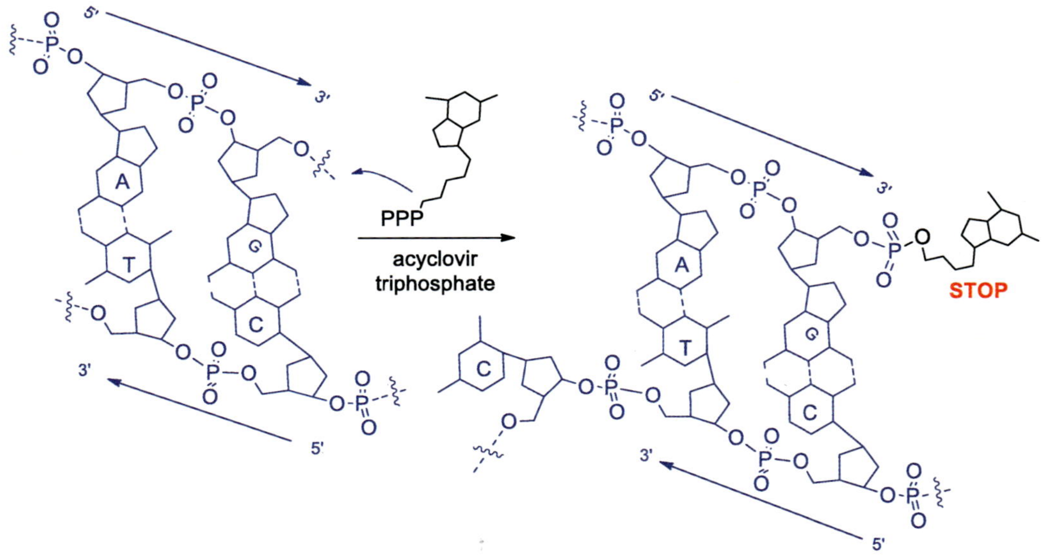

The drug Vidarabine, (adenine-arabinoside), a synthetic analog to deoxyadenosine, has the same mechanism of action as that of acyclovir and is useful to treat various human herpes viruses. Acyclovir is preferred over Vidarabine since the latter causes low white blood cell counts and neurotoxicity [31c-d].

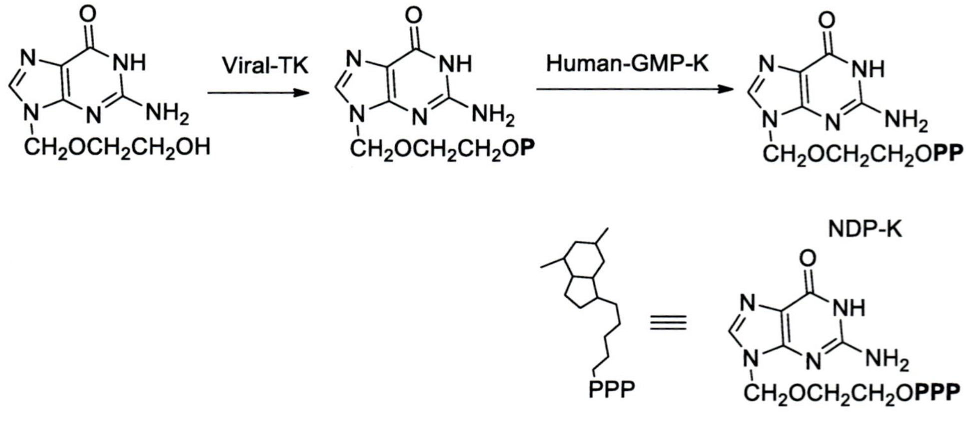

Synthesis

This is prepared by N^9-alkylation of guanine with the chloromethyl ether [2-(chloromethoxy)ethyl propionate] followed by saponification [31h].

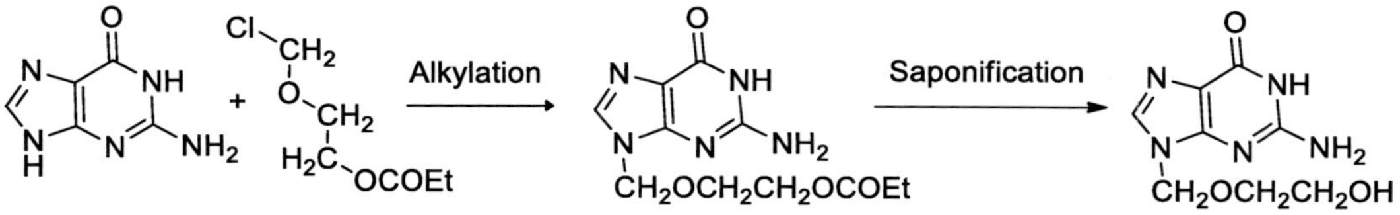

Guanine on treatment with (2-acetoxyethoxy) methyl acetate in acetic anhydride as a solvent and in the presence of *p*-toluenesulfonic acid as a catalyst results in two isomeric mixtures (9/7) of diacetylacyclovir in the 1:45 ratio. The mixture is then concentrated and heated under reduced pressure, which results in the mixture (9/7-isomer) in the 17:1 ratio. Treatment with ethyl acetate and acetonitrile produced pure 9-isomer. The acetylated product is then hydrolysed and acidification results in a cyclovir [31h].

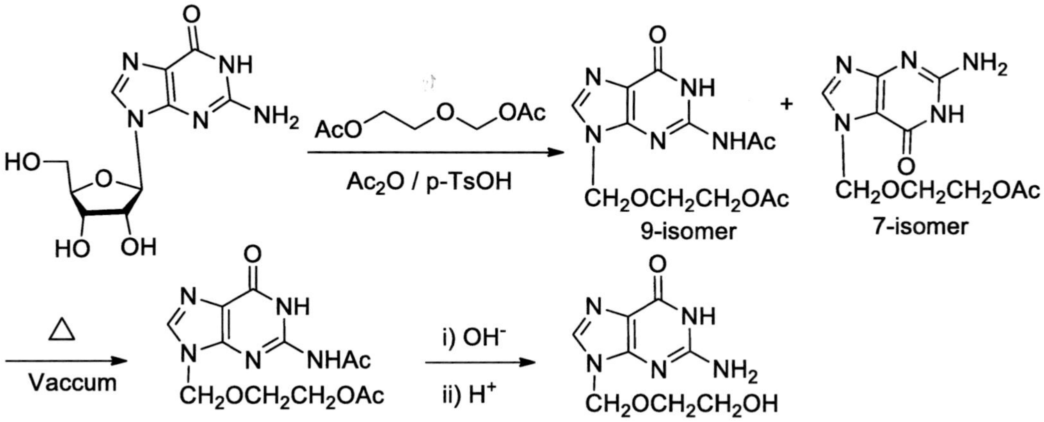

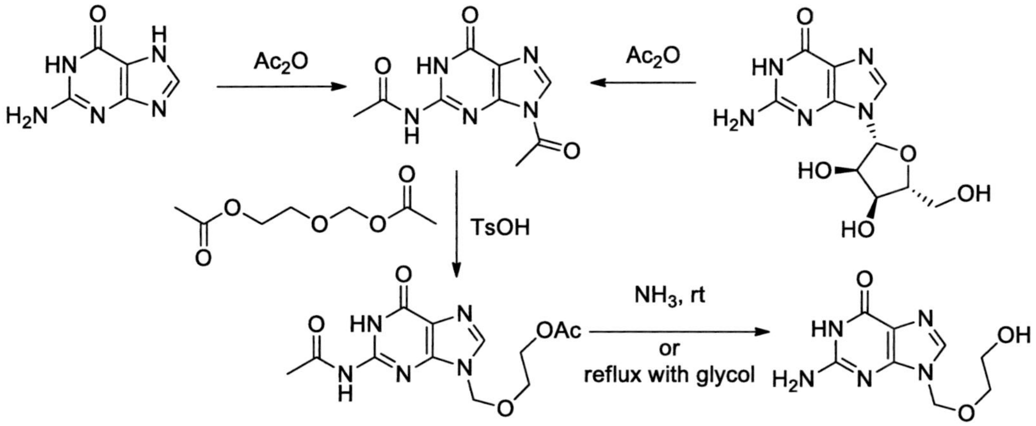

The acetylation of the guanine base or guanosine nucleoside gives the diacetyl guanine. Diacetylated guanine is condensed with 1,4-diacetoxy-2-oxabutane in the presence of 4-methylbenzenesulfonic acid (TsOH) to yield N,O-diacetyl acyclovir. Finally, deacetylation gives acyclovir.

Synthesis of acyclovir is done from benzoyl chloride, which is treated with ethylene glycol in the presence of the amine base to give ethylene glycol monobenzoate. This could also be achieved from benzonitrile with refluxing ethylene glycol. This is chloromethylated with formaldehyde and dry HCl in CH_2Cl_2 to give 1-benzoyloxy-2-chloromethoxyethane. The condensation of guanine with refluxing hexamethyldisilazane followed by reaction with 1-benzoyloxy-2-chloromethoxyethane in the presence of triethylamine with refluxing benzene gives 9-(2-benzoyloxyethoxymethyl) guanine. The product is finally hydrolyzed with ammonia in methanol at 80 °C in a pressure vessel to give acyclovir.

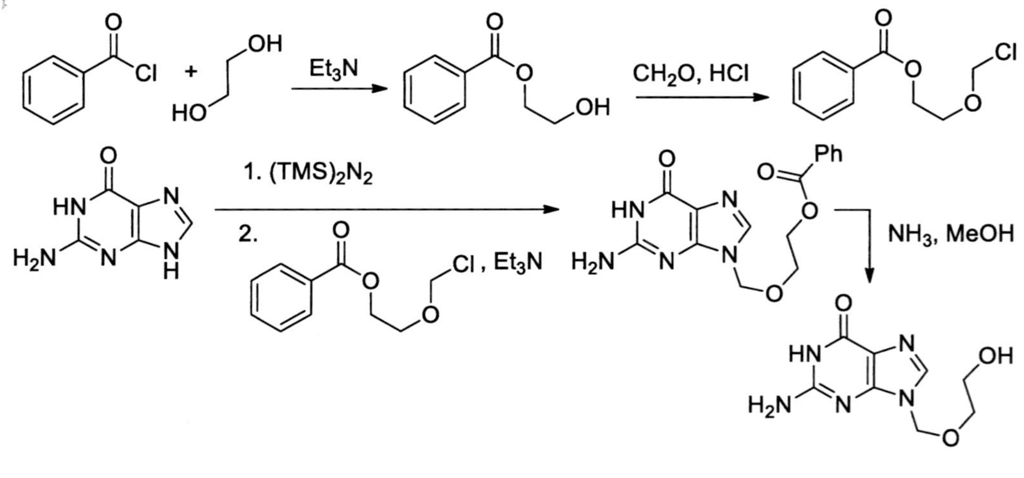

The condensation of 1-benzoyloxy-2-chloromethoxyethane with 2,6-dichloropurine in the presence of the amine base like triethylamine in DMF yields 2,6-dichloro-9-(2-benzoyloxyethoxymethyl)purine. The product is selectively aminated and debenzoylated by treatment with NH_3 in methanol at 95 °C in a pressure vessel to give 2-chloro-9-(2-hydroxyethoxymethyl)adenine. The Sandmeyer reaction of aromatic amine results in 2-chloro-9-(2-hydroxyethoxymethyl) hypoxanthine. Finally, ammonolysis with ammonia in methanol at 125 °C in a pressure vessel replaces chlorine to give acyclovir [31h].

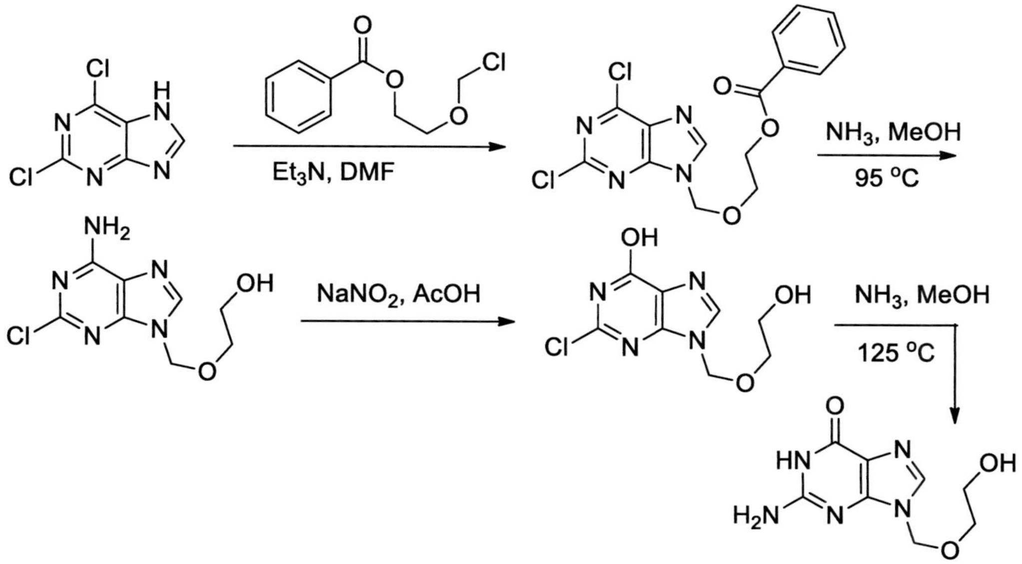

An efficient and selective process for the synthesis of acyclovir has also been reported by the reaction of guanine with refluxing hexamethyldisilazane (HMDS) and trifluoromethanesulfonic acid (TFA). Excess HMDS is eliminated and subsequent reflux with 1,3-dioxolane gives the product 9-[2-(trimethylsilyloxy) ethoxymethyl]guanine which on hydrolysis with acetic acid-water under refluxing condition gives acyclovir [31h].

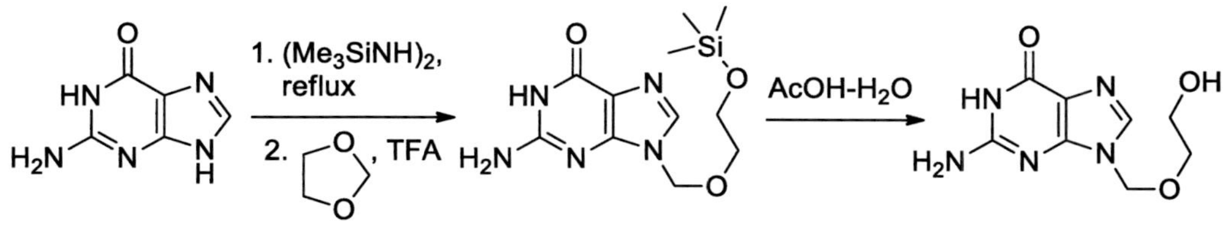

HIV-AIDS RELATED DRUGS

AZT- Zidovudine

Zidovudine (ZDV), thymidine nucleoside analogue (dideoxynucleoside) reverse-transcriptase inhibitor (NRTI), is an example of antiretroviral medication used to prevent and treat Acquired Immune Deficiency Syndrome (AIDS) caused by Human Immunodeficiency Virus (HIV) in humans. It has a high affinity to an enzyme called reverse transcriptase than DNA polymerase used for human cell division, which is used by retroviruses such as HIV to replicate viral single-stranded RNA (ribonucleic acid) into proviral double-stranded DNA (deoxyribonucleic acid). It is also known as azidothymidine (AZT). Zidovudine was first used in the United States in 1987 under the brand name Retrovir® [13-15]. This is used both orally and in injection form. It is commonly used in pregnancy to prevent mother-to-child spread during birth. The common side effects of this medicine are nausea, vomiting, headache, dizziness, fatigue, weakness, muscle pain, lactic acidosis, liver problems, myopathy, and blood disorders resulting in anemia and leukopenia.

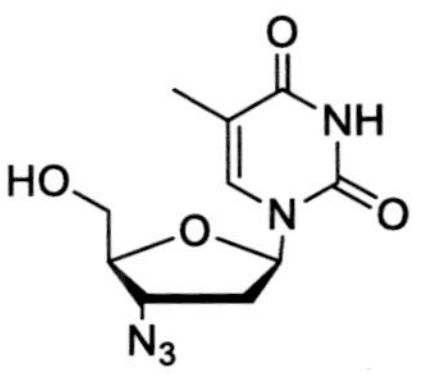

1-((2*R*,4*R*,5*S*)-4-azido-tetrahydro-5-(hydroxymethyl)furan-2-yl)-5-methylpyrimidine-2,4(1*H*,3*H*)-dione

(Zidovudine)

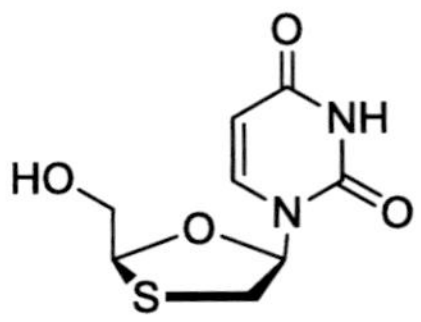

Lamivudine (3TC)

A retrovirus (*e.g.*, HIV) is a virus that contains core RNA. Retrovirus is duplicated in a host cell using the reverse transcriptase enzyme to create DNA from its RNA [5]. The synthesized DNA can transcribe RNA and direct protein synthesis. In zidovudine, the 3'-hydroxy group on the sugar moiety is replaced by an azido group. This prevents the nucleic acid chain growth (DNA replication) at the 3'-position of the sugar by a phosphodiester linkage. This ultimately acts as a chain-terminator of viral DNA during reverse transcription.

Lamivudine, also called 3TC, is another cytosine nucleoside analogue and contains deoxyribose sugar [13, 15, 17]. Lack of the hydroxyl group prevents and treats HIV/AIDS. In the reverse transcription process, nucleoside gets incorporated into the DNA chain. But due to the lack of the hydroxyl group, the addition of a nucleotide to the DNA chain will be stopped. Lamivudine is useful for AZT-resistant viruses and used in combination with AZT-drug effectively.

Synthesis

Functionalisation of Thymidine Moiety

DEAD (diethyl azodicarboxylate) or DIAD (diisopropyl azodicarboxylate) assists thymidine transformation to the intramolecular ether derivative. The ether easily converts to zidovudine when treated with azide, followed by basic hydrolysis [32d, 17].

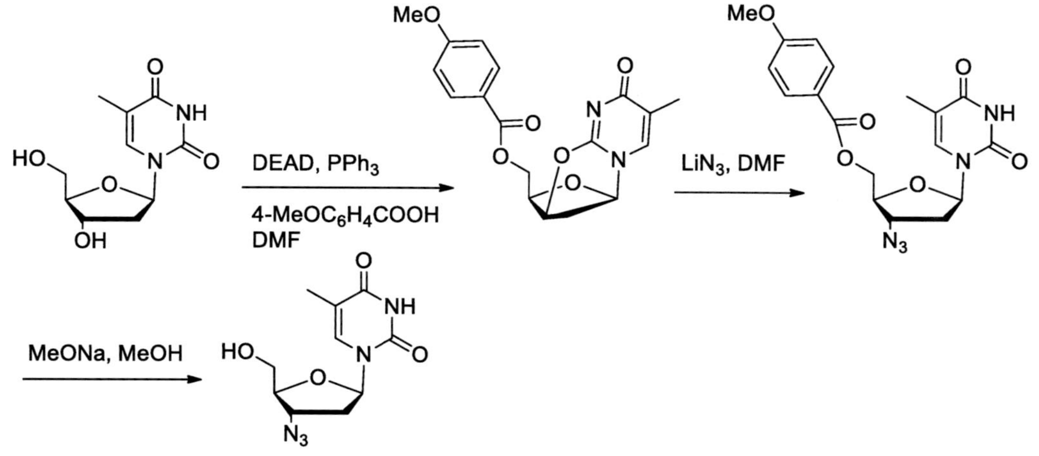

This intramolecular cyclic-ether like bond is also made from 5'-*O*-tritylthymidine. 5'-*O*-tritylthymidine is mesitylated with mesyl chloride and is cyclized using potassium phthalimide in hot DMF water. This results in 5'-*O*-trityl-2,3'-anhydro-thymidine and subsequent reaction with sodium azide in refluxing DMF - water gives 5'-*O*-trityl-3'-azido-3'-deoxy thymidine. Now deprotection with 80% aqueous acetic acid gives AZT [32e].

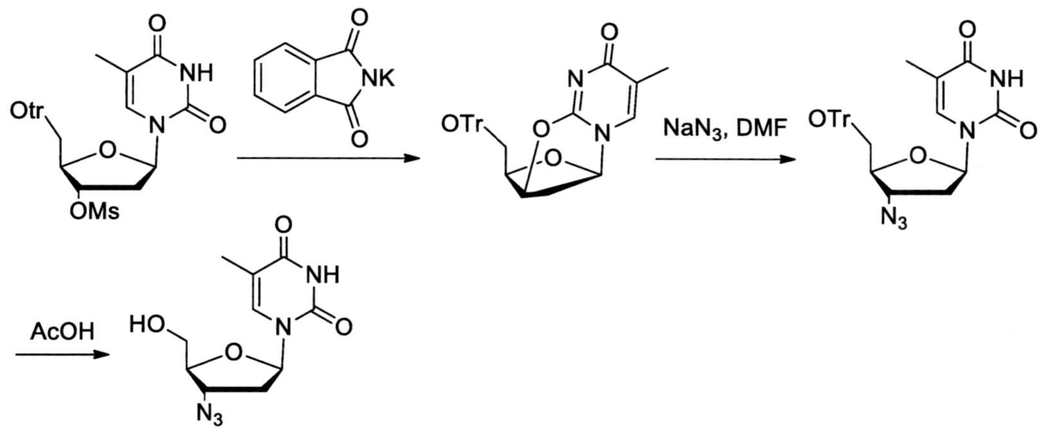

Building of Furanose Moiety

This involves D-mannitol as the starting material. D-mannitol, on protection and oxidation, results protected glyceraldehydes. The pentan-2-enal derivative is obtained *via* vinylogation at low temperature and fluoride assisted deprotection of O-Si bond. Azidation results azido-aldehyde, which is treated with $TiCl_4$ and subsequent coupling with thiamine derivative results AZT [32a].

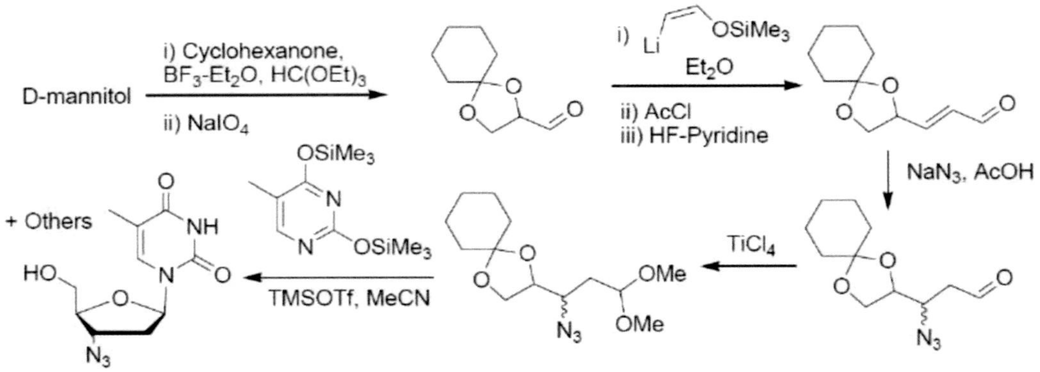

In another case, *cis*-3-(2,2-dimethyl-1,3-dioxolanyl)-propan-2-enoate on hydrolysis gives 5-(hydroxymethyl)furan-2(5H)-one which on silyl-ether protection and azide-Michael addition gives azido-lactone. *Cis*-3-(2,2-dimethyl-1,3-dioxolanyl)-propan-2-enoate is easily synthesized from D-mannitol *via* oxidative degradation and Horner–Wadsworth–Emmons (HWE) reaction. Lactone is reduced to lactol selectively by DIBAL and then amide coupling with thiamine derivative results in TBDMS protected zidovudine. Deprotection of silyl ether using fluoride results in zidovudine [32].

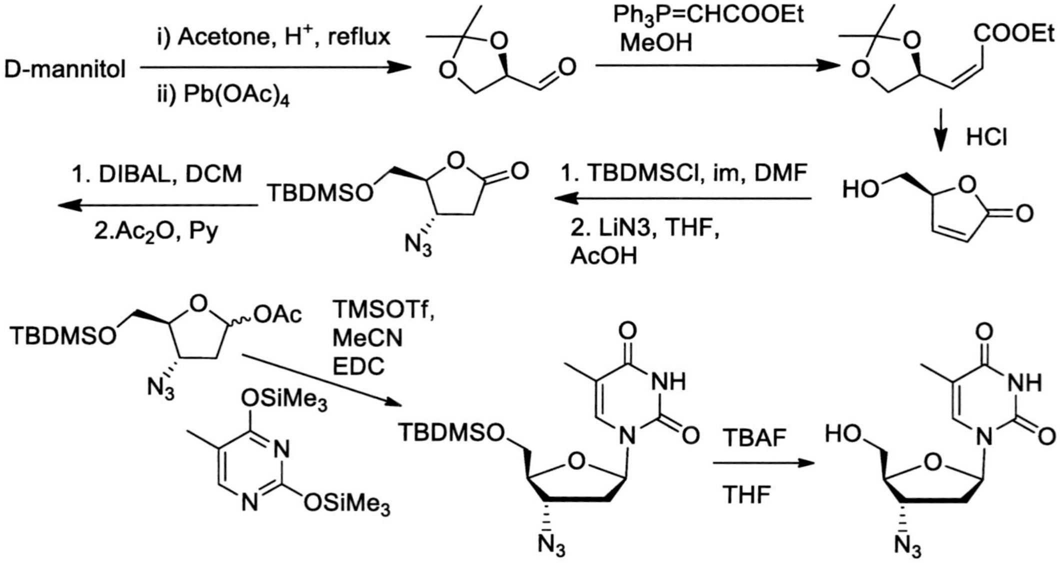

CHAPTER 5

Drugs and Pharmaceuticals: Retrosynthetic Analysis

Abstract: In this chapter, basic retrosynthetic approach has been introduced. Rretro-synthetic analysis of some common drugs *e.g.* Aspirin, Paracetamol, Ibuprofen, Chloroquin, Primaquine, Norfloxacin, Fluconazole, Dapsone, Sulphonamides, Sulfamethoxazole, Sulphacetamide, Trimethoprim have been shown here with justifications.

Keywords: Drug discovery, Pharmaceuticals, Pharmaceutical chemistry, Pharmacology, Pharmacokinetics.

BASIC RETROSYNTHETIC APPROACH

Retrosynthesis is important in order to answer the best synthetic route of a target molecule from available or all possible route [33, 34]. The best synthetic route must have certain criteria, *i.e.*, shorter synthetic route, minimum waste, cost-effective, better yield, available starting materials and reagents, easiest reaction condition, *etc.*

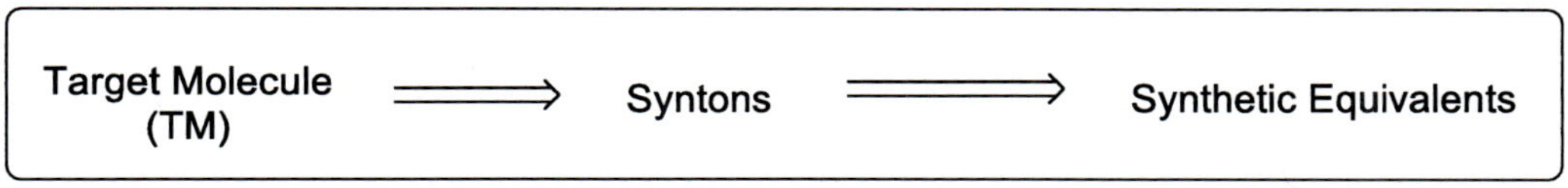

The main aim of the retrosynthetic analysis is to find out the best synthetic route for the desired molecule, called the target molecule. Transform involves the reverse of a synthetic reaction, the formation of starting materials from a single product. The main transforms are disconnections & functional group interconversions (FGI).

Disconnection

The reverse process of a reaction (approach) involves the breaking of a bond to form possible starting materials. This involves at least two synthons [7, 33].

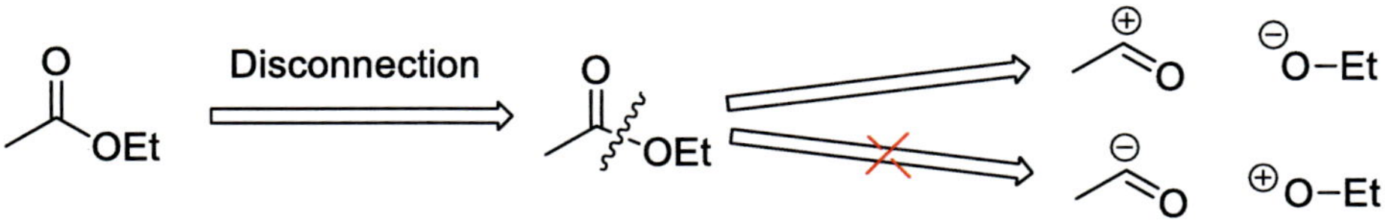

Functional Group Interconversions(FGI)

The reverse process of a reaction that converts one functional group into another by substitution, elimination, oxidation and reduction reaction is known as Functional Group Interconversions (FGI) [7, 33]. This involves one synthon with addition/elimination of hetero-atom mainly but not with C.

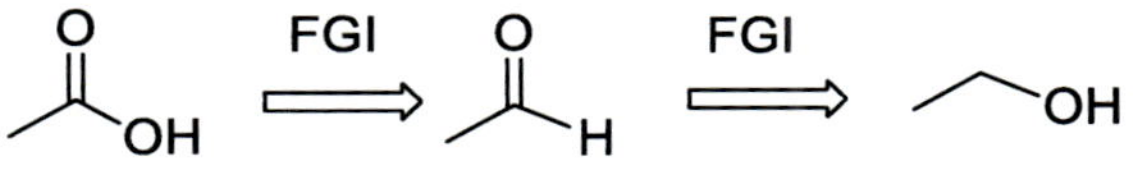

Synthon

It is the fragments of the target that results from breaking a bond heterolytically. This may or may not be important for the synthesis of the TM [33].

Acylcation 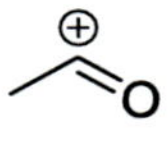 is synthon (Imaginary Part of the target) for ethyl acetate.

Synthetic Equivalent

The actual substrates used for the forward synthesis are the synthetic equivalent. Acetyl chloride is asynthetic equivalent (commercially available) [33].

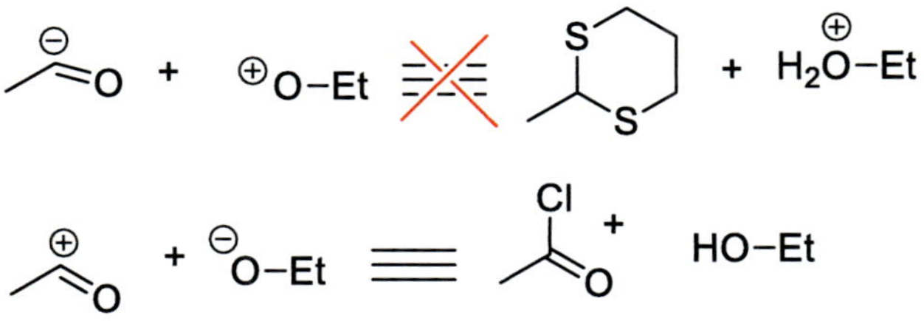

Donor and Acceptor Synthons

Synthon that behaves as electrophile is acceptor synthon, and the synthon that behaves as a nucleophile is donor synthon [33].

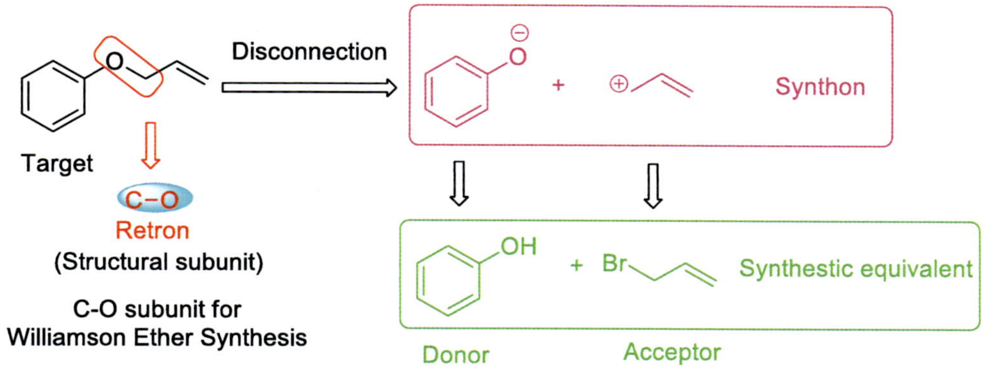

Retron

A minimal molecular substructure that enables certain transformations is known as retron [33]. Synthesis of ether requires minimal structural units like O-H and C-X bond whatever ether you are going to synthesize.

In a retrosynthetic analysis, it is advised to disconnect the molecule near to heteroatom or nearby bond. Therefore, all possible disconnection may not be good at the point of synthesis. In the given example, path b is more acceptable for its easy reaction condition.

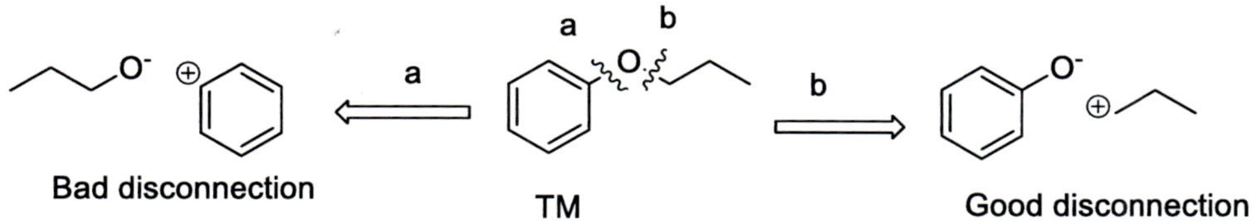

It is also important to think in such a way so that *umpolung* is avoided until or unless it is mandatory since this requires either less easily accessible starting materials or harsh reaction conditions [33].

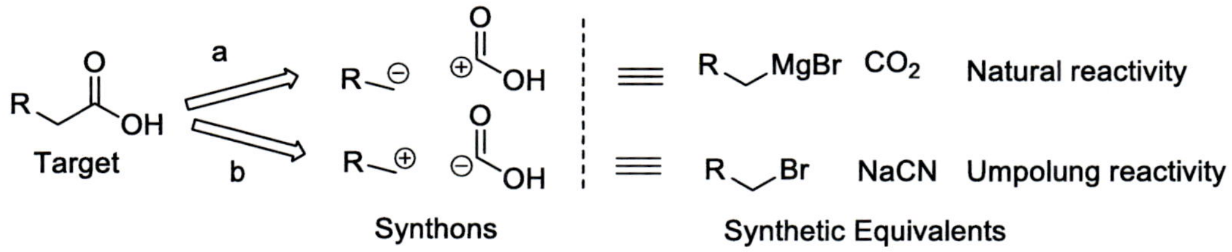

Example

For acylation of the aminophenol, amine undergoes acylation faster if the Ph-OH is unionised. Therefore,the reaction is not better in alkaline conditions. Thus, the following analysis is acceptable and synthesis.

Retrosynthetic Analysis

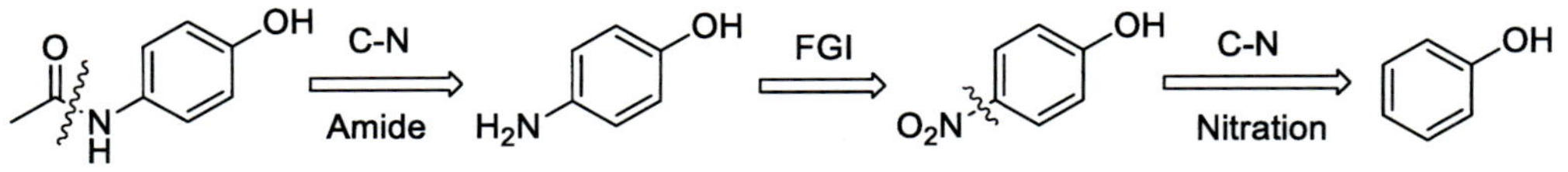

Synthesis

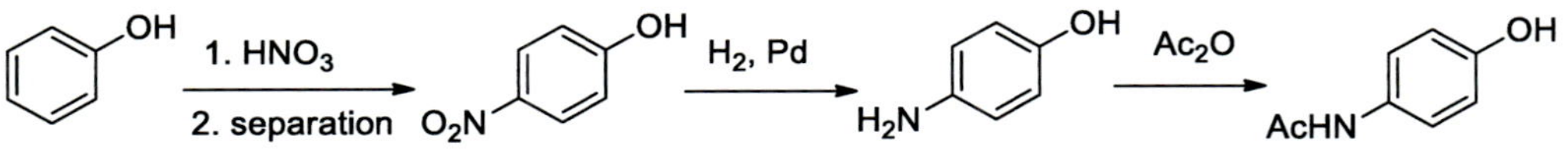

RETRO-SYNTHETIC ANALYSIS OF SOME COMMON DRUGS

Aspirin

It is easy to recognize two starting equivalent of aspirin, *e.g.*, aceyl equivalent and phenolic equivalent. Salicyclic acid gives phenol part, and either acetic anhydride or acetyl chloride gives aceyl equivalent [7].

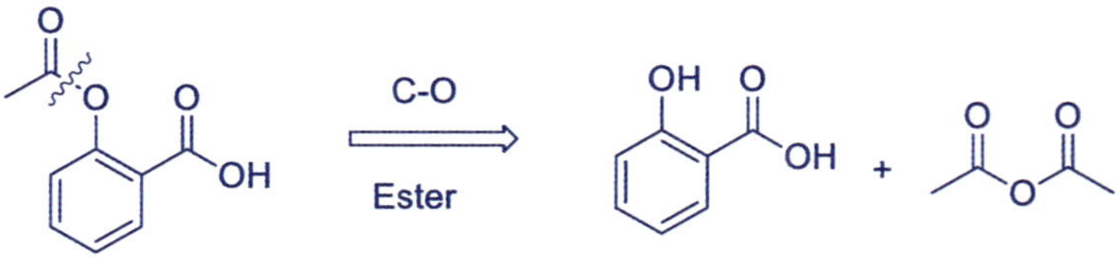

Chemical synthesis of aspirin is achieved in the old days using salicylic acid and acetic anhydride. But recently, acetyl chloride is the open choice for many reasons.

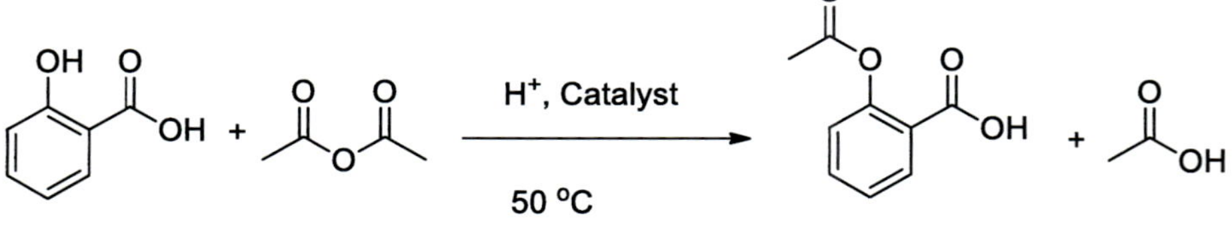

Paracetamol

Paracetamol can be disconnected into *para*-aminophenol and acetyl chloride or acetic anhydride (acetyl equivalent). According to the functional group interconversion of (FGI) of *para*-aminophenol, the precursor is *para*-nitrophenol [7].

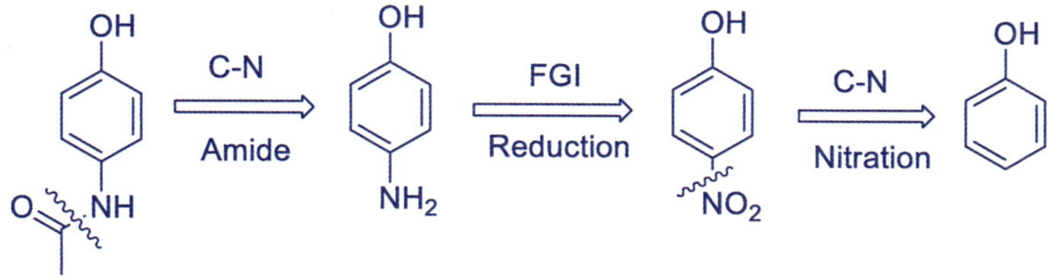

Based on the retrosynthetic analysis, acetyl chloride or acetic anhydride would be the ideal reagent for synthon $MeCO^+$. But the best choice of reagent is acetic anhydride. The byproduct acetic acid is easier to handle than HCl.

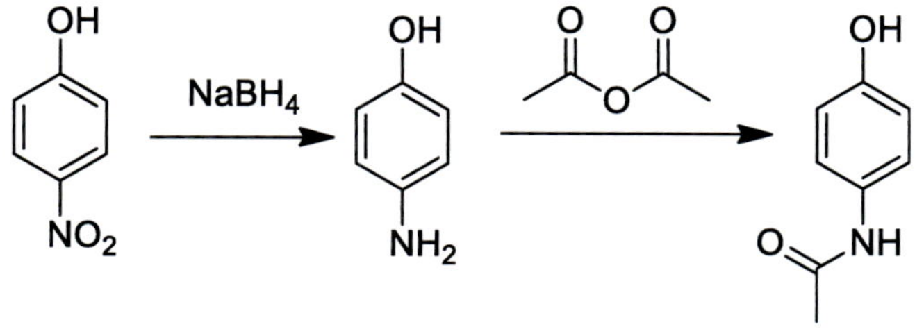

In another way, it can be disconnected into *p*-hydroxyacetophenone after converting the functional group (FGI) into oxime. *p*- hydroxyacetophenone is then further disconnected into cheap and available material phenol [7].

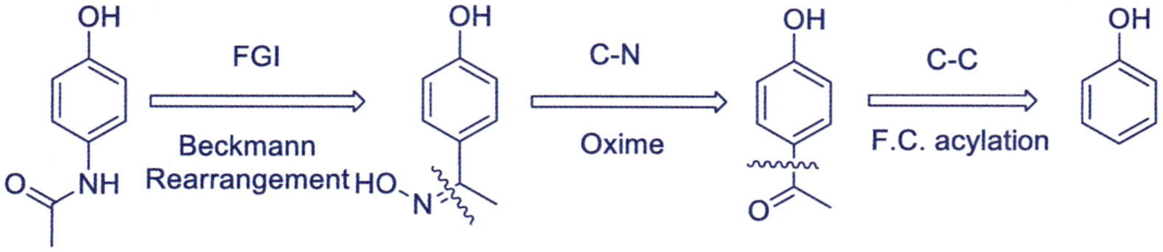

Phenol is easily transformed into *p*-hydroxyacetophenone *via* Fridel-Craft aceylation. Ketone is then converted to oxime, which on Bechmann rearrangement, results paracetamol.

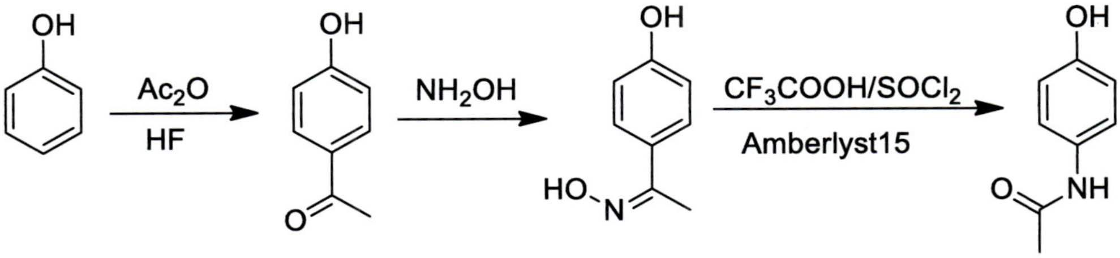

Ibuprofen

Functional group interconversion (FGI) of acid gives cyanide. Another functional group inter-conversion (FGI) of cyanide gives oxime. Double bonded C-N disconnection resulted in the aldehyde. To get synthetic equivalent isobutylbenzene as starting material, C-C disconnection of the aldehyde has to be set up such that it came from acetophenone unit [33].

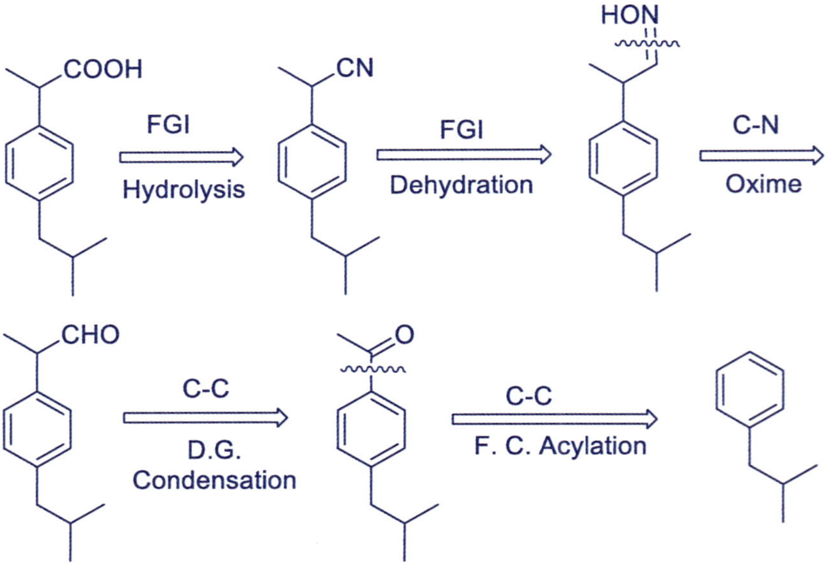

Therefore, in the forward synthesis, Fridel-Craft aceylation of isobutylbenzene gives *p*-acetyl substituted molecule. Now, Darzenglycidic ester synthesis followed by hydrolysis will be the perfect sequence to desire aldehyde. Aldehyde can easily be transformed into acid *via* numerous processes to get ibuprofen.

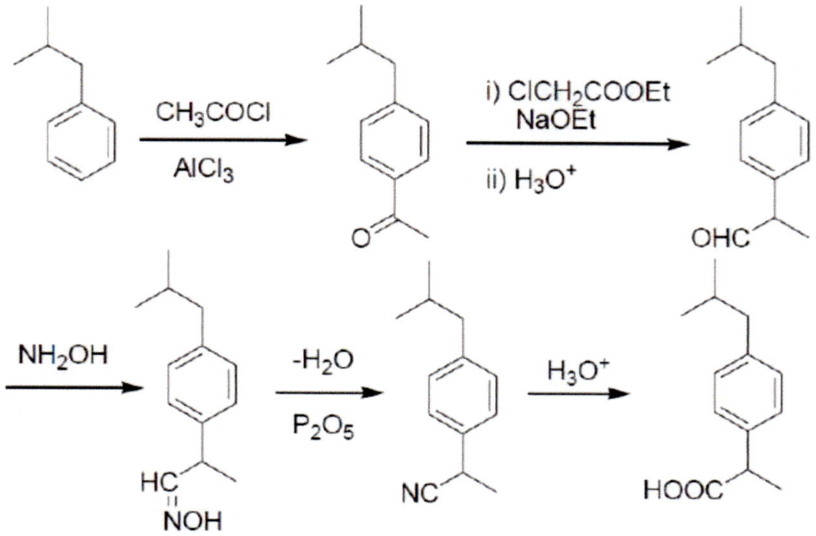

One-step conversion of alcohol into acid is effective when the Pd- catalysed carbonylation step is introduced. Therefore, ibuprofen is disconnected into the 1-phenylethanol derivative. Functional group interconversion (FGI) gives an easy synthetic equivalent that could be prepared from the Fridel-Craft aceylation method from isobutylbenzene [33].

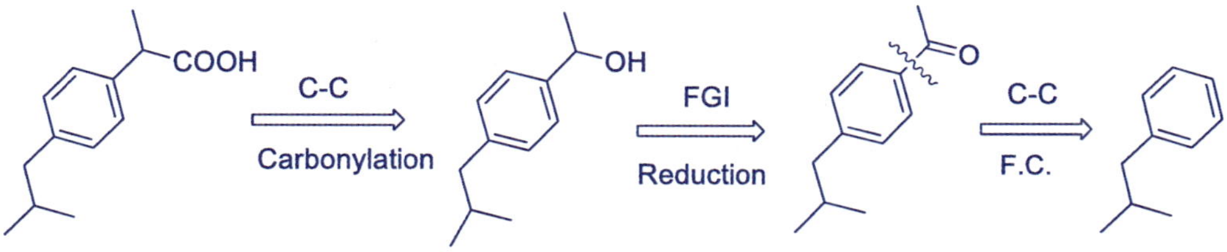

Extra steps in the Boot method have been modified by Hoechst–Celanese methods using the Pd-c catalysed carbonylation step. This avoided too many steps with byproducts. They use 3-catalytic steps with high atom economy.

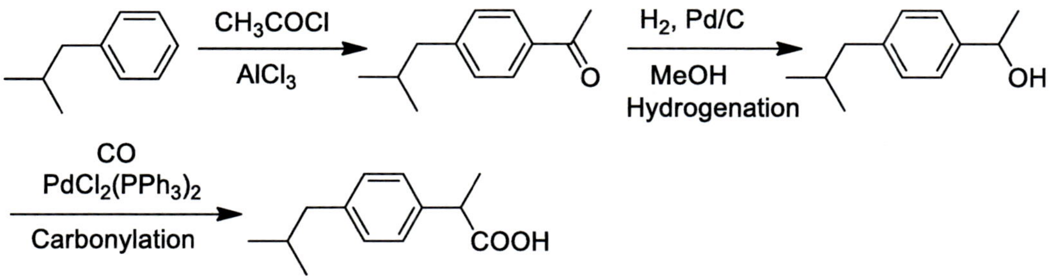

Benzylic metalations of the aromatic compound and sequential alkylation are expected to be good to find C-C bond disconnection. The same metalation technique may be useful for carbonylation.

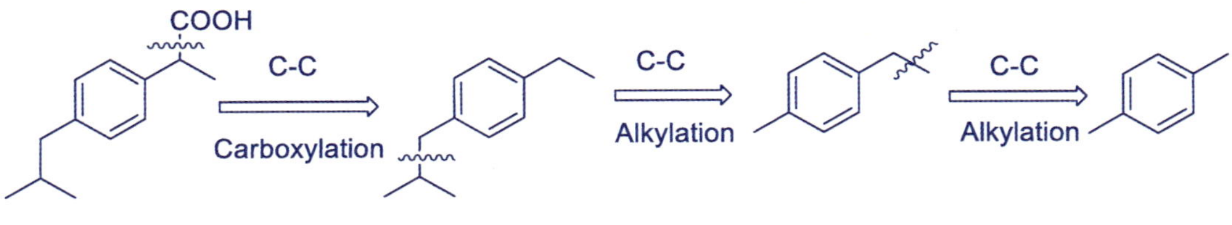

In the forward synthesis, alkylation resulted in ethyl-*p*-isobutylbenzene. More acidic benzylic proton is removed off to install carboxylate ion.

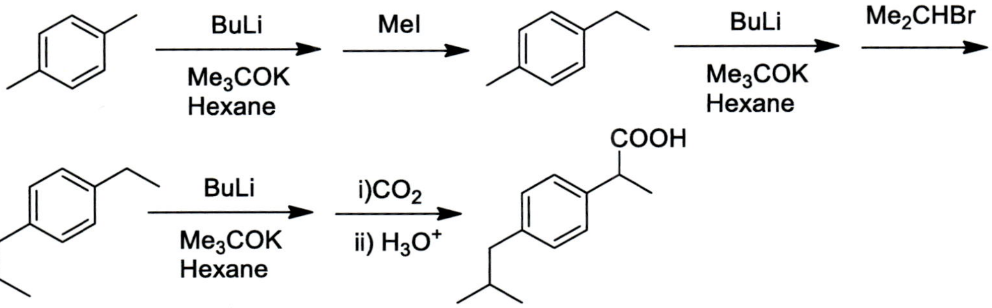

Chloroquine

Side chain of the aromatic compound with C-N retron is straight-forwardly disconnected considering nucleophilic substitution reaction. Therefore, the proper substrate for C-N bond disconnection is an aromatic halide. This can be accessed on functional group inter-conversion (FGI) to form phenol like substrate. At this stage, functional group addition (FGA) is important so that C-C bond disconnection will be appropriate considering condensation from 1,3-dicarbonyl compound [33]. This 1,3-dicarbonyl compound is disconnected considering the C-N coupling reaction from m-chloroaniline and diethyl 2-(ethoxymethylene)malonate as synthetic equivalents.

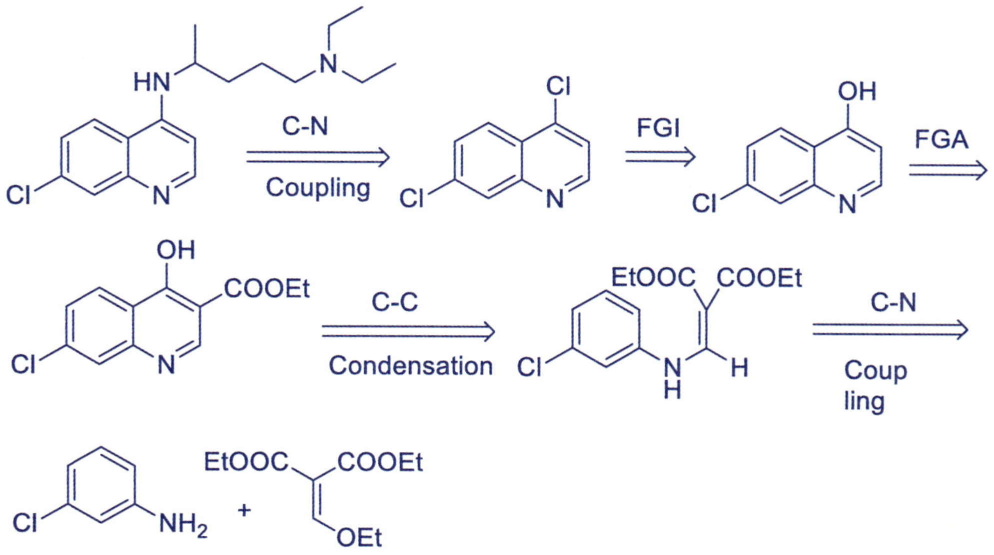

In the forward synthesis, *m*-chloroaniline and diethyl 2-(ethoxymethylene) malonate are heated to condensed to get 1,3-dicarbonyl compound in good yield. 7-chloroquinolin-4-ol is the key intermediate that is accessible *via* the aromatic cyclisation process. The functional group inter-conversion (FGI) of hydroxyl to chloro then gives the proper substrate for C-N coupling with N_1,N_1-diethylpentane-1,4-diamine [33].

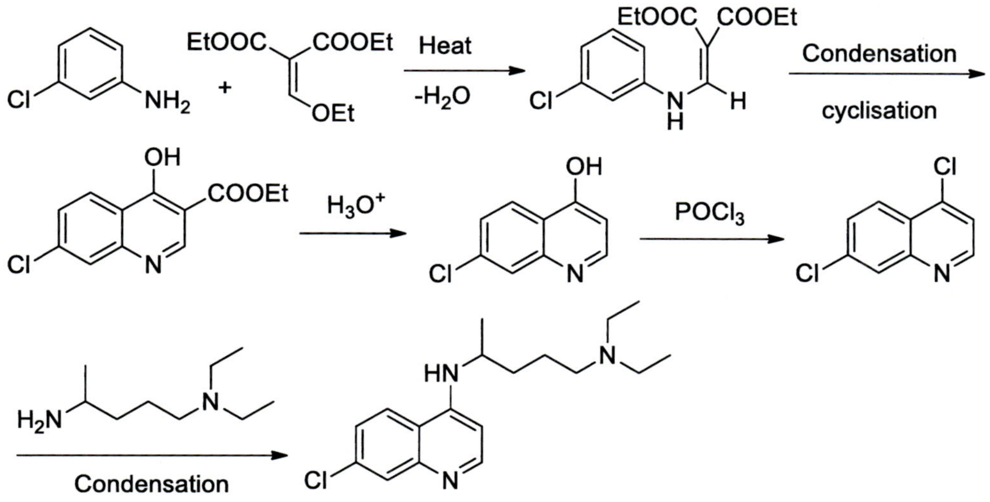

Primaquine

It is always considered a part of amine group synthesis in a protected manner. Otherwise, the alkylation is challenging due to the greater reactivity of the product amine. Therefore, in the retrosynthetic analysis, the amine group is masked as phthalimide group after functional group addition (FGA) [33]. The C-N bond of phthalimide is disconnected to get the two synthetic equivalents. Another disconnection of the C-N bond helps to find the starting dibromo-compound.

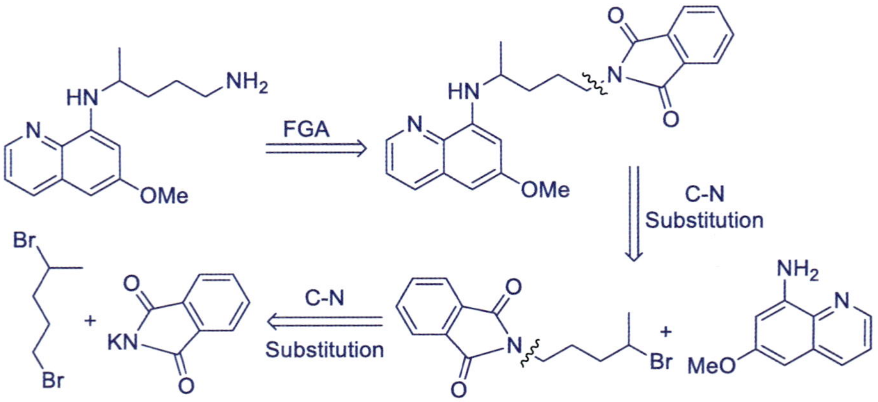

Therefore, consecutive N-alkylation followed by hydrolysis resulted in amine compound from masked amine. In the early step, primary alkyl halide reacts preferably with phthalimide than the secondary amine at ambient condition but higher energy is needed for alkylation of aromatic amine.

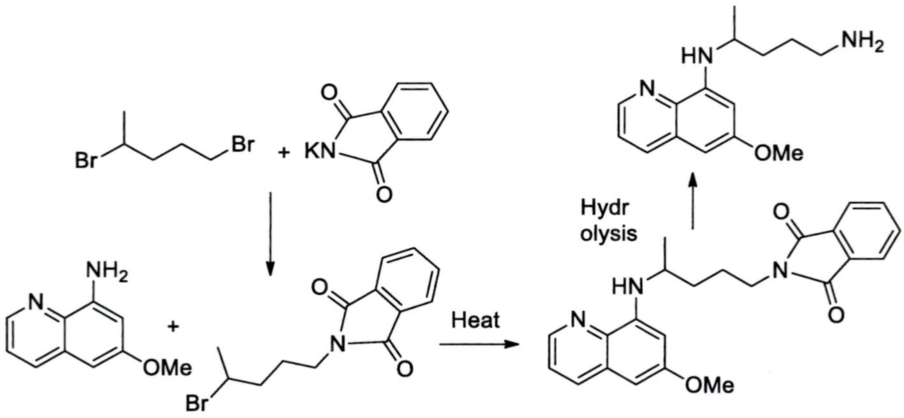

Norfloxacin

Norfloxacin clearly indicates the presence of 4-quinolinone with few substitutions. Retrosynthetic analysis of this requires disconnection of C-N bonds and then synthesis of 4-quinolinone. The first disconnection requires a C-N bond of piperazine unit, and the second one is an N-substituted ethyl group. Then two-step disconnection of C-C and C-N bonds gives 3-chloro-4-fluoroaniline and diethyl 2-(ethoxymethylene)malonate considering cyclisation-condensation reaction.

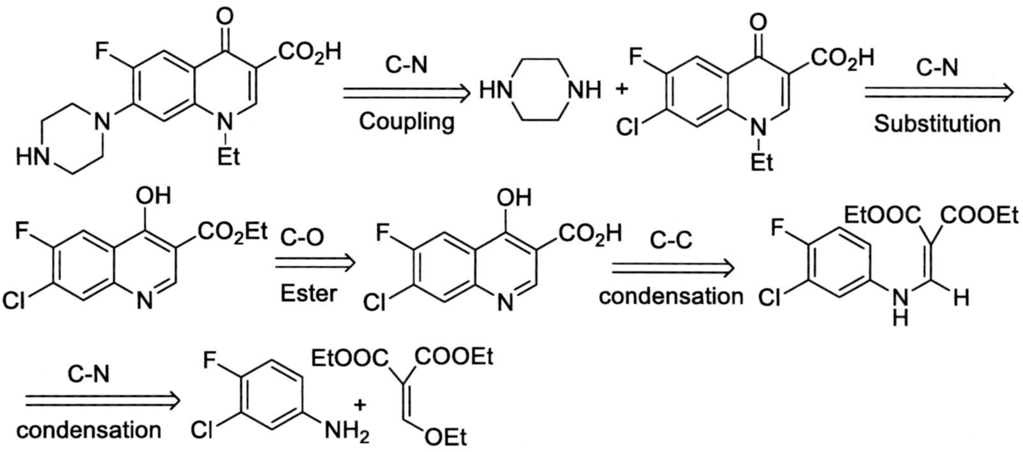

In the forward synthesis, step-wise condensation-cyclisation gives 4-quinolinone skeleton, and then step-wise C-N bond formation gives the target molecule.

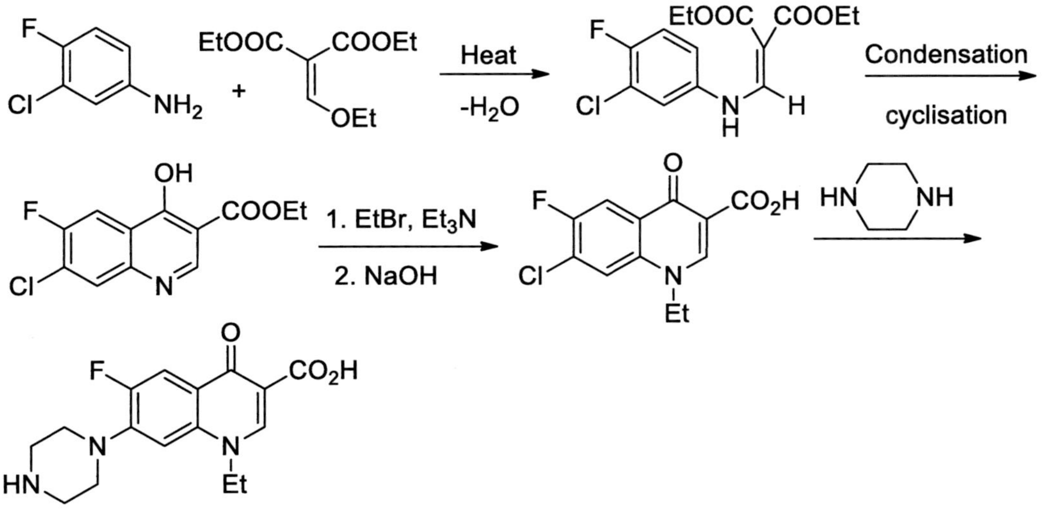

Fluconazole

The fluconazole has two 1,2,4-triazole units. The analysis supports the introduction of one unit by substitution with α-chloro-acetophenone moiety and the second one *via* epoxy ring-opening. Thus, 1, 2-diX disconnection results epoxide [33]. This epoxide is disconnected considering carbene-like insertion reaction. The C-N disconnection of mono 1,2,4-triazole substituted acetophenone gives α-chloro-acetophenone. Further C-C disconnection gives commercially available 1,3-difluorbenzene and chloroacetyl chloride.

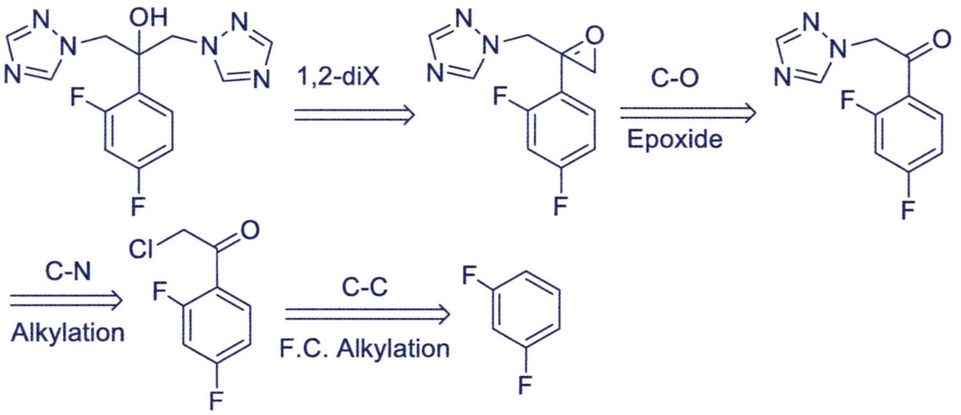

1,3-difluorbenzene under Fridel-Craft acylation with chloroacetyl chloride gives α-chloro-difluoroacetophenone. The C-N bond is developed *via* the substitution reaction with 1,2,4-triazole. Corey-Chaykovsky reaction is very useful to construct epoxide from carbonyl moiety. Regioselective ring opening by nitrogen nucleophile of 1,2,4-triazole allows to form the second 1,2,4-triazole unit in fluconazole.

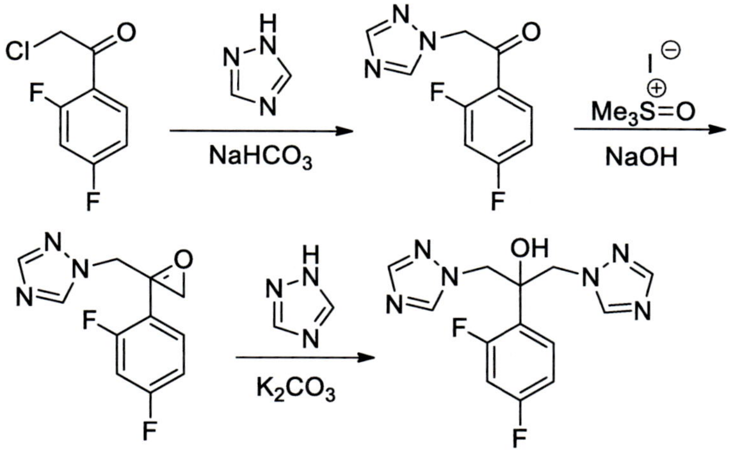

Dapsone

Di-(*p*-aminophenyl) sulfone unit is usually inter-converted into corresponding d*i*-(*p*-nitrophenyl) sulfone and then into d*i*-(*p*-nitrophenyl) sulfide. The sequence of inter-conversion of the functional group is important here. Disconnection at C-S hetero bond gives the synthetic equivalent *p*-chloronitrobenzene [6, 33].

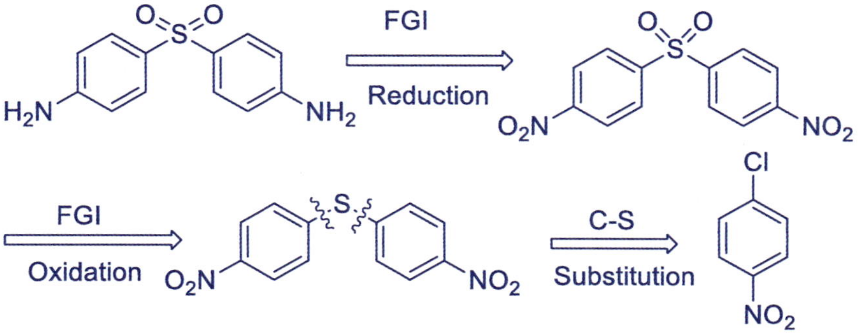

Aromatic nucleophilic substitution of *p*-chloronitrobenzene with sodium sulfide easily results di-(*p*-nitrophenyl) sulfide. Oxidation gives sulfone, and then reduction of nitro-group gives dapsone.

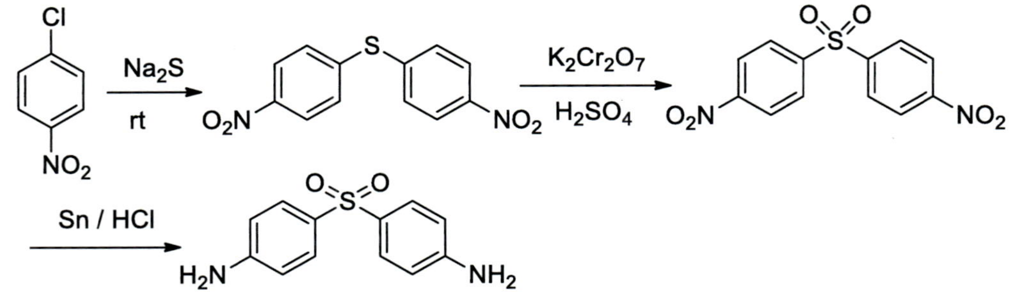

Di-phenyl sulfone is also used as a synthetic equivalent for di-(*p*-nitrophenyl) sulfone. di-phenyl sulfone is produced by the sulfonation of benzene with sulfuric acid and oleum.

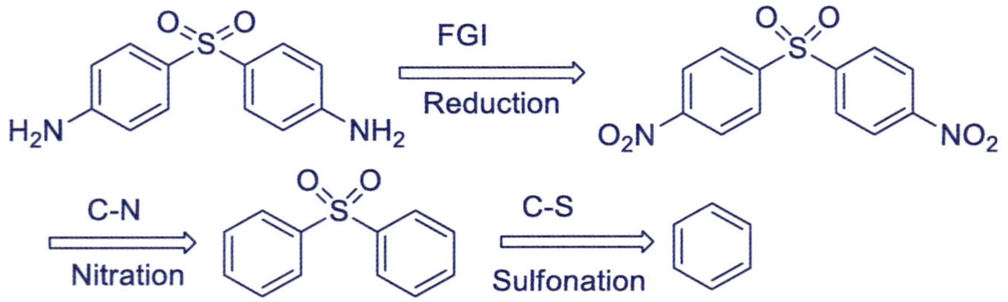

Therefore, sequential sulfonation, nitration and reduction are used as another synthetic route for dapsone.

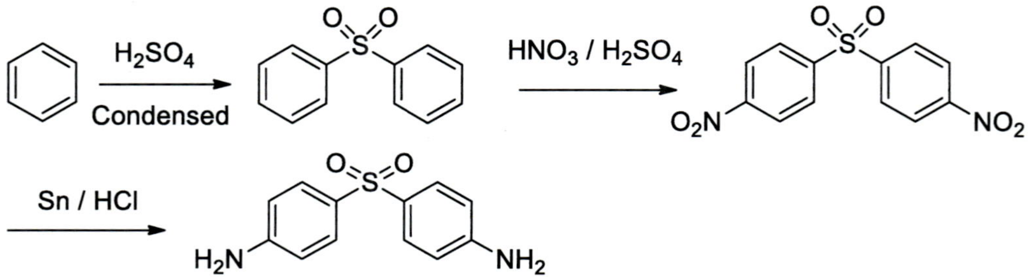

Disconnection of the C-S bond of sulfone gives a synthetic equivalent arylsulfinate and *p*-chloronitrobenzene considering the aromatic nucleophilic substitution reaction. Arylsulfinate must be chosen properly as the amine group competes with the reaction.

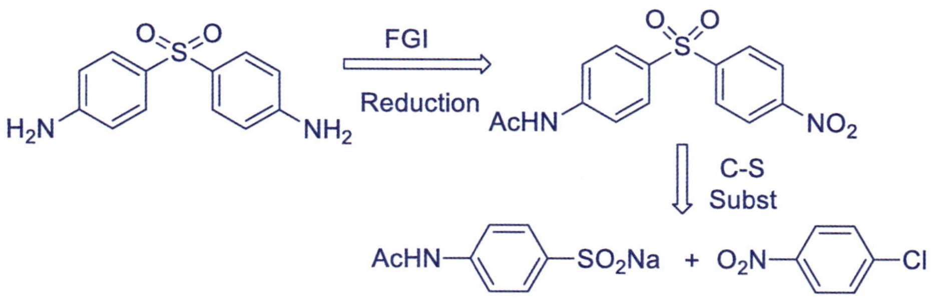

Sodium 4-acetamidobenzenesulfinate is considered the nucleophile for the aromatic nucleophilic substitution reaction with *p*-chloronitrobenzene followed by hydrolysis results dapsone.

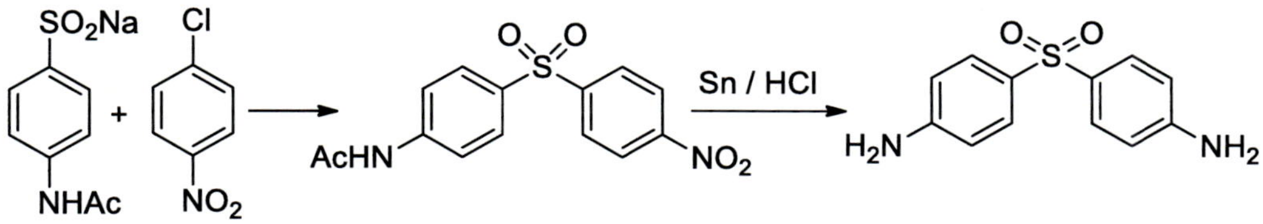

Sulphonamides

For the strong electronic effect of aniline, the direct introduction of chloro sulfonyl group is ineffective which is why, reactivity is reduced before the Friedel-Craft reaction. Functional group interconversion of an amine into amide and sulfonamide into chloro sulfonyl group gives the synthetic equivalent 4-acetamidobenzene-1-sulfonyl chloride.

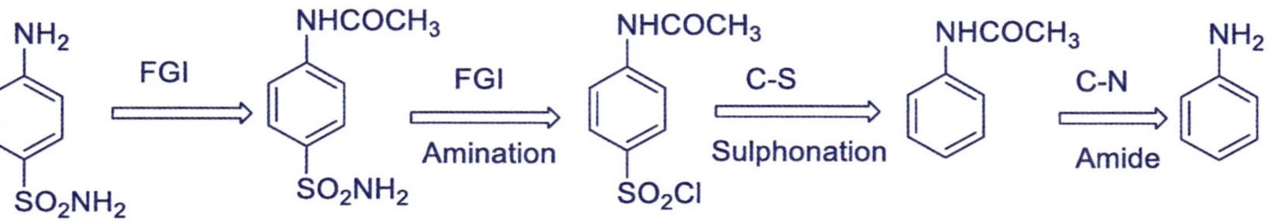

Thus, amine is protected with an acetyl group, and then chloro sulfonyl group is introduced. Amination and hydrolysis effectively result in sulphonamide [6].

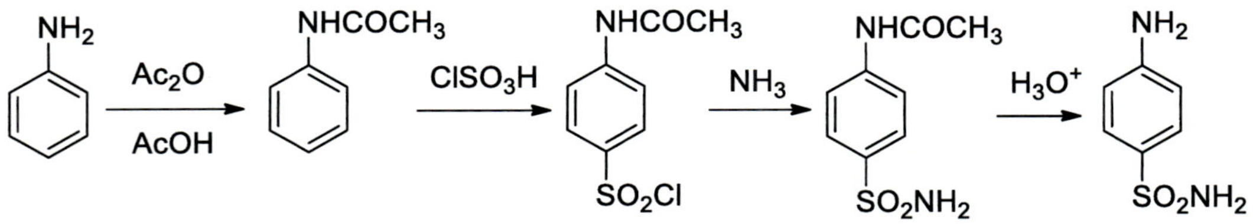

Sulphanethoxazol

Disconnection of sulphamethoxazole at S-N bond gives easily accessible two structural units of 5-isoxazol and aryl sulfonyl chloride. Aryl sulfonyl chloride is interconverted to 4-acetamidobenzene-1-sulfonyl chloride.

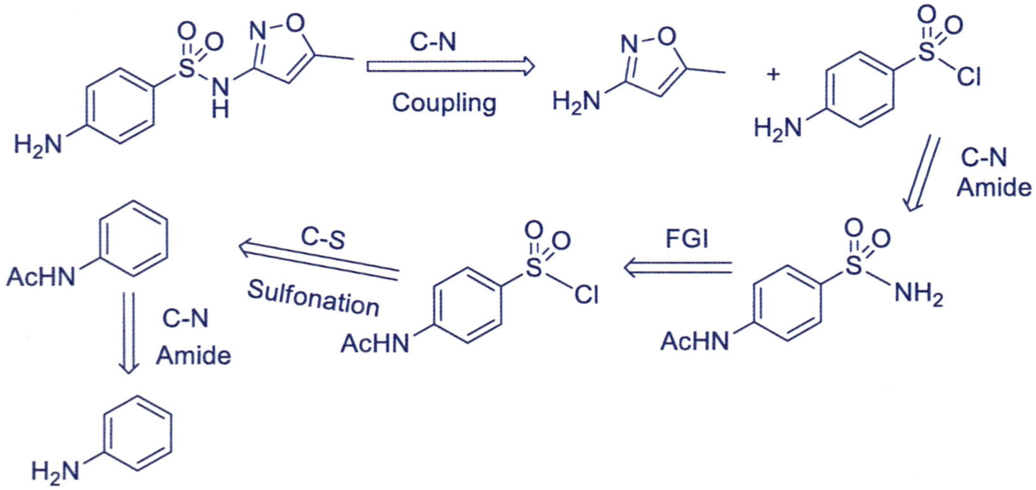

However, simple synthetic equivalents are obtained by disconnecting the S-N bond.

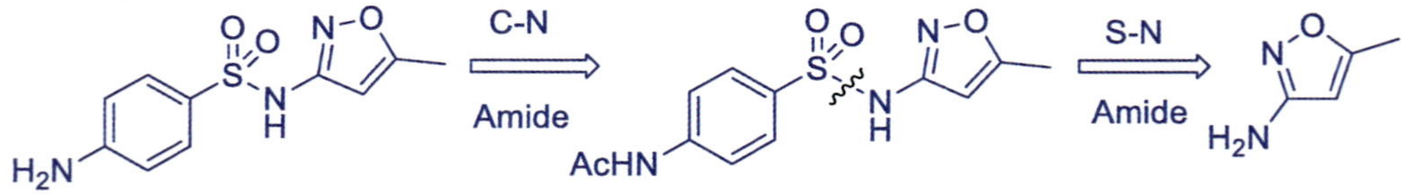

Amide bond formation of amino isoxazole with aryl sulfonyl chloride seems to be the easiest way to get sulphanethoxazol.

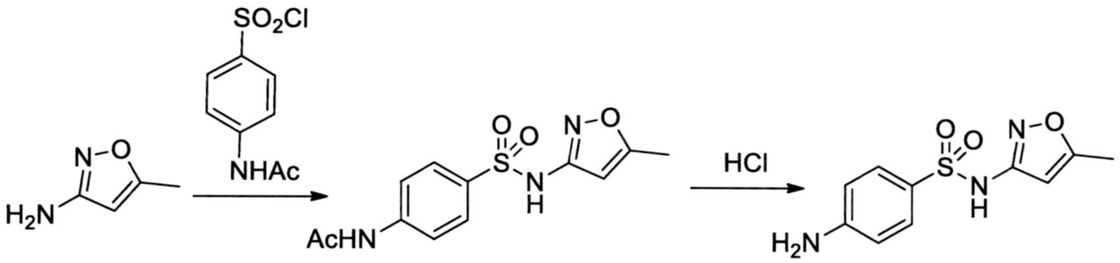

Sulphacetamide

The structure of sulphacetamide is indicative for disconnection at S-N bond to consider aryl sulfonyl chloride and acetamide as starting materials [6].

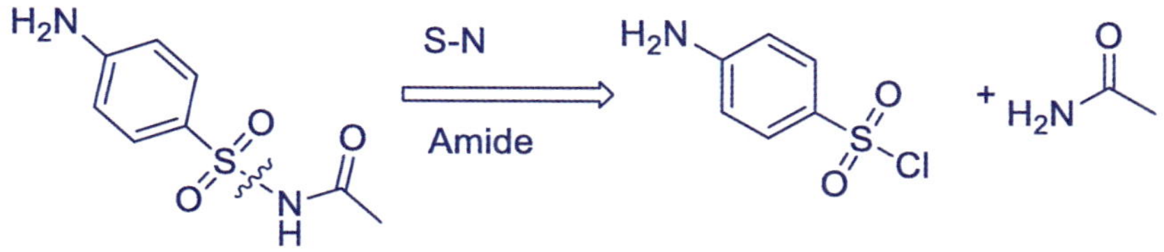

Either of aryl sulfonyl chloride or sulfonamide isa useful substrate for the N-(arylsulfonyl)acetamide. The use of acetic anhydride is considered as best due to the formation of acetic acid as a byproduct, however availability matter.

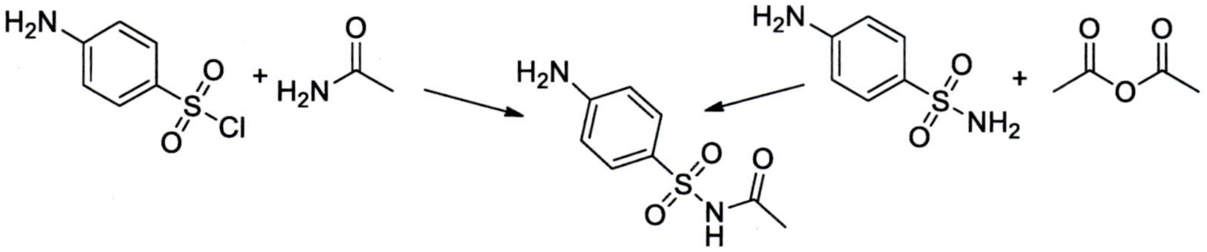

Commercially available aniline is converted into 4-acetamidobenzene-1-sulfonyl chloride for sulfonamide. Amine group of sulfonamide is protected, and then selective hydrolysis gives N-((4-aminophenyl)sulfonyl)acetamide.

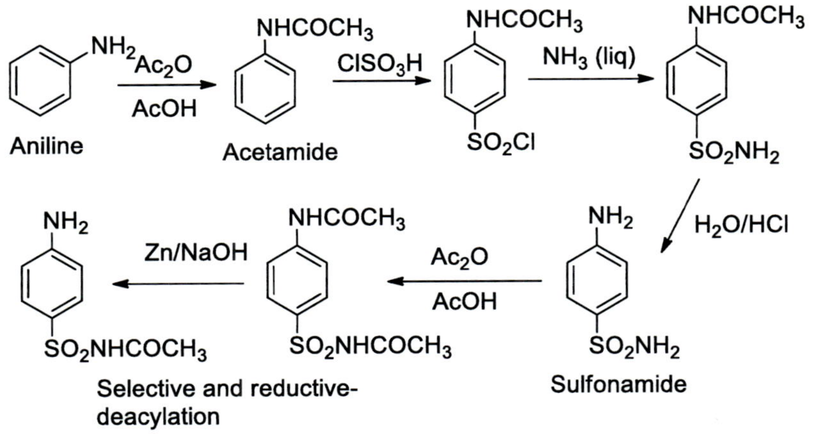

Trimethoprim

The usual disconnection of trimethoprim is the C-N bonds of the pyrimidine ring and gives guanidine as one of the synthetic equivalents. Another one is the 1,3-carbonyl compound in which two functional groups are at 1,3-position, which can be disconnected as 1,3-diCO [33].

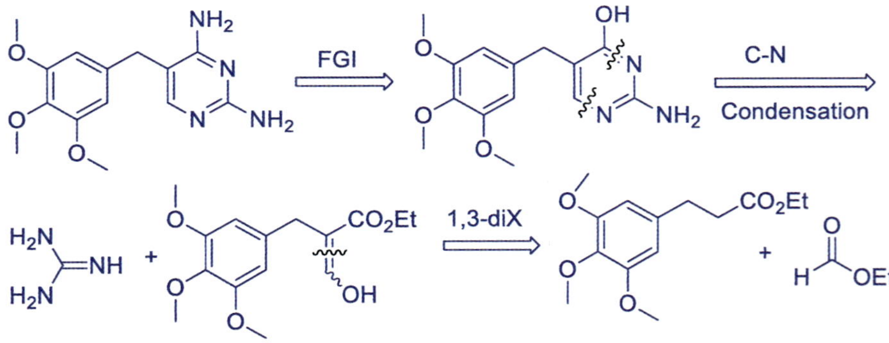

Formylaton of the 3-arylpropanoate results in 1,3-dicarbonyl compound. The 1,3-dicarbonyl compound is condensed with guanidine to get the pyrimidine framework. The reaction of hydroxypyrimidine with phosphorous oxychloride and then amination gives trimethoprim.

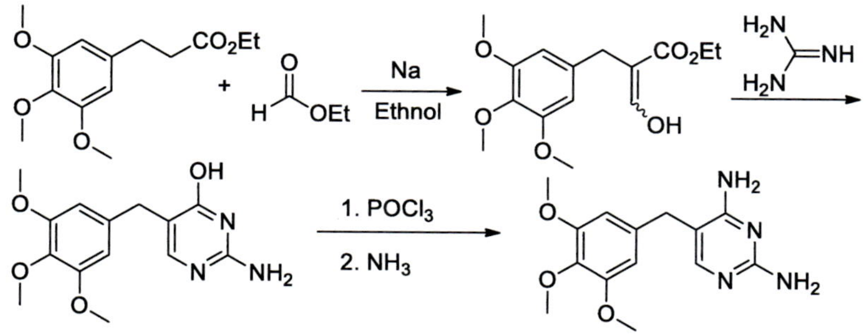

Disconnection of trimethoprim could also give α-substituted-β-aminoacrylonitrile. This is further disconnected at C-C bond for nucleophilic substitution with trimethoxybenzyl cation as a synthon.

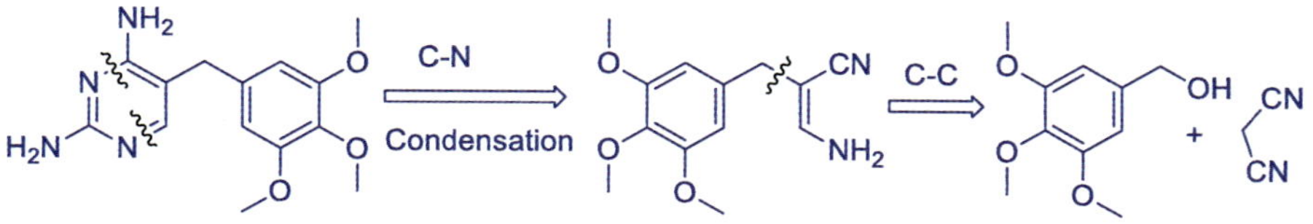

In the forward synthesis, trimethoxybenzyl alcohol acts as an electrophile in the presence of malononitrile. Substitution reaction gives α-substituted-β-aminoacrylonitrile. Condensation of guanidine with this furnishes trimethoprim.

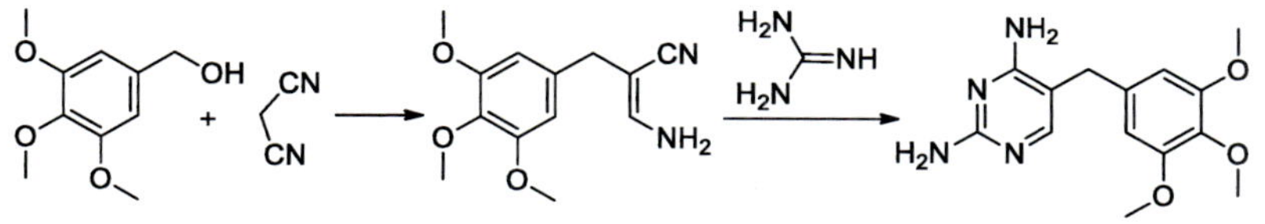

MORE EXAMPLES

Chloramphenicol

Retrosynthetic Analysis 1

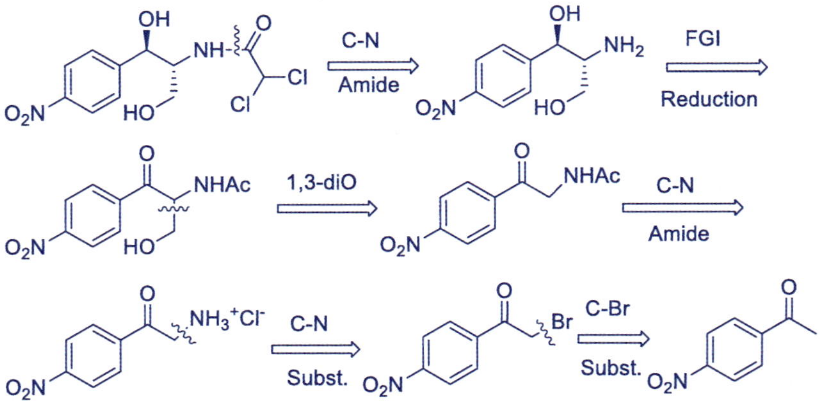

Chemical Synthesis 1

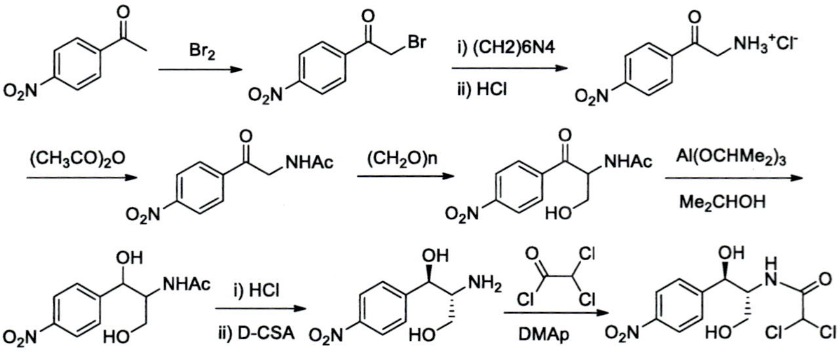

Retrosynthetic Analysis 2

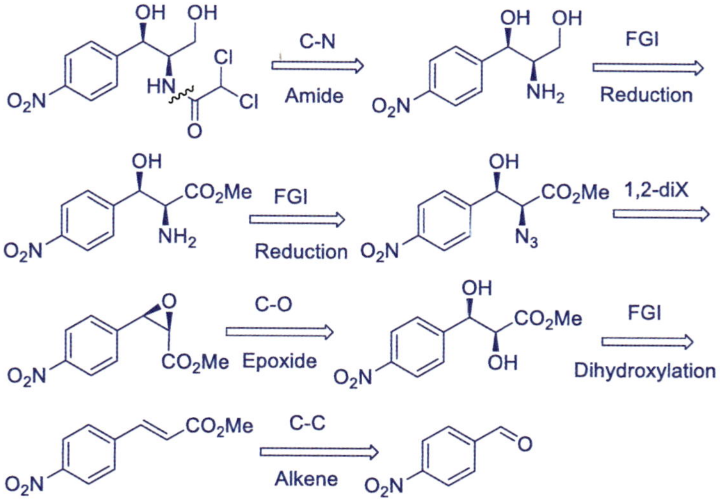

Chemical Synthesis 2

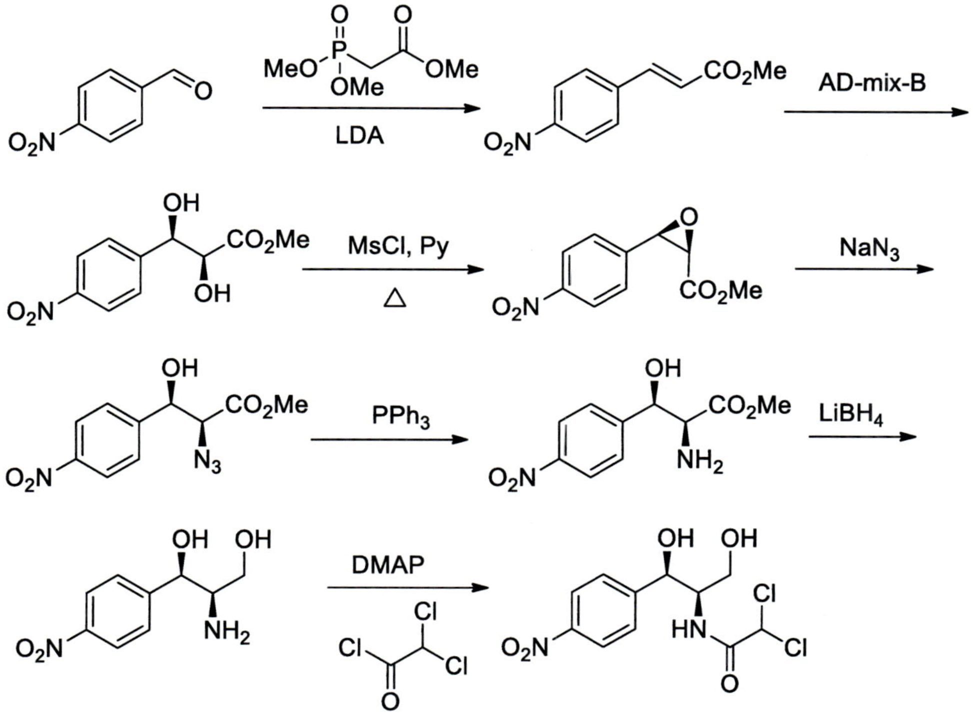

Trimethoprim

Retrosynthetic Analysis 1

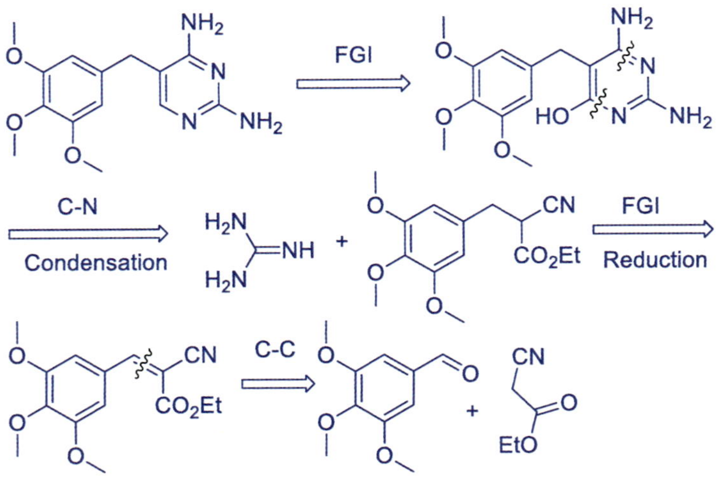

Chemical Synthesis 1

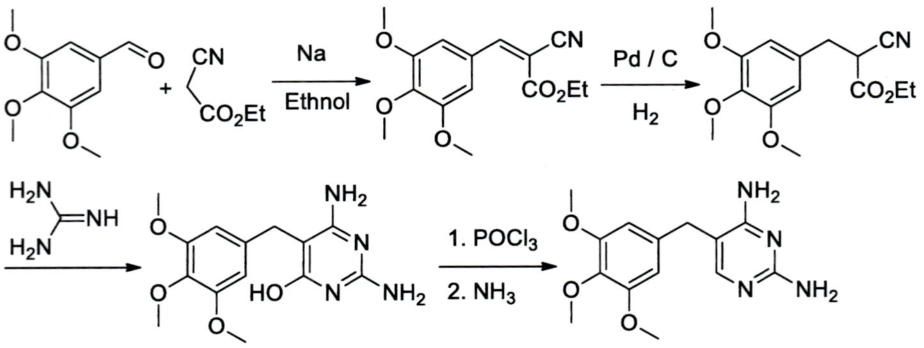

Retrosynthetic Analysis 2

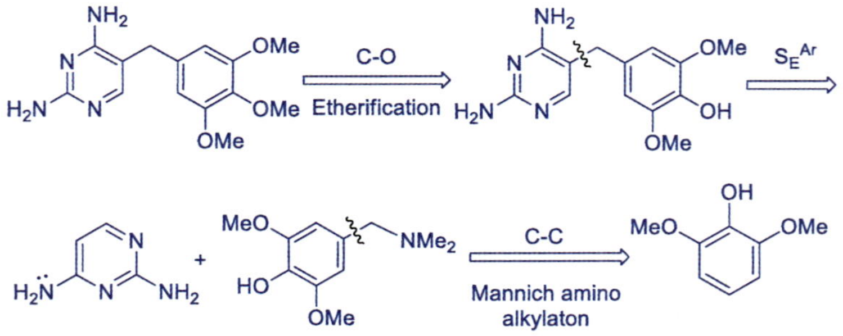

Chemical Synthesis 2

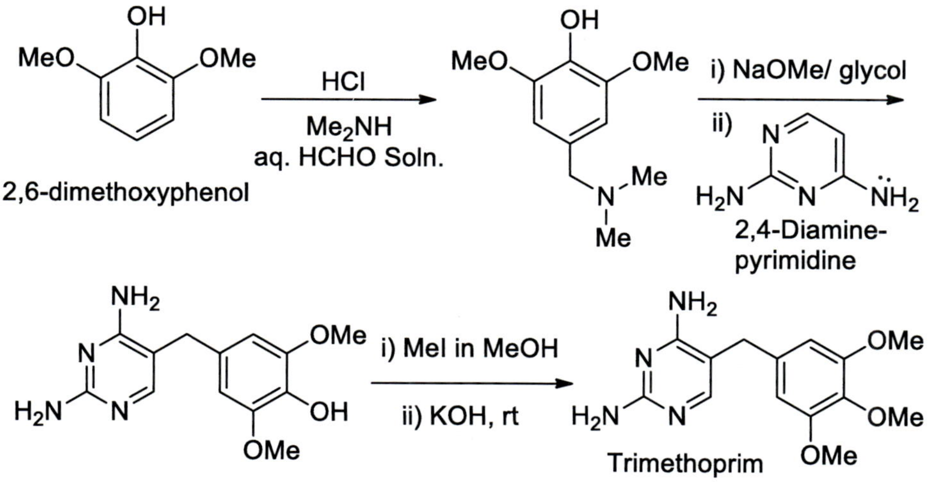

Acyclovir

Retrosynthetic Analysis 1

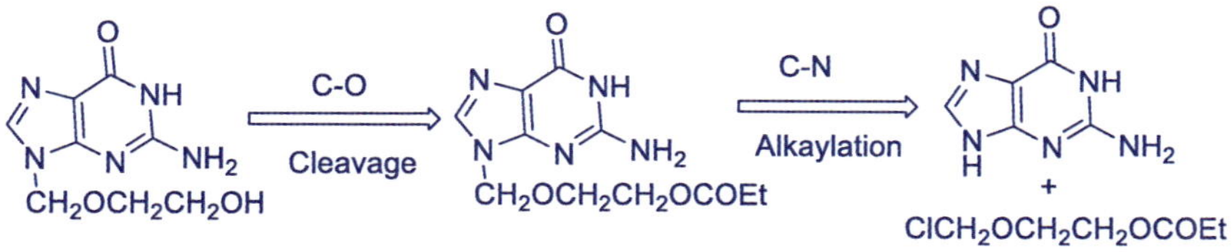

Chemical Synthesis 1

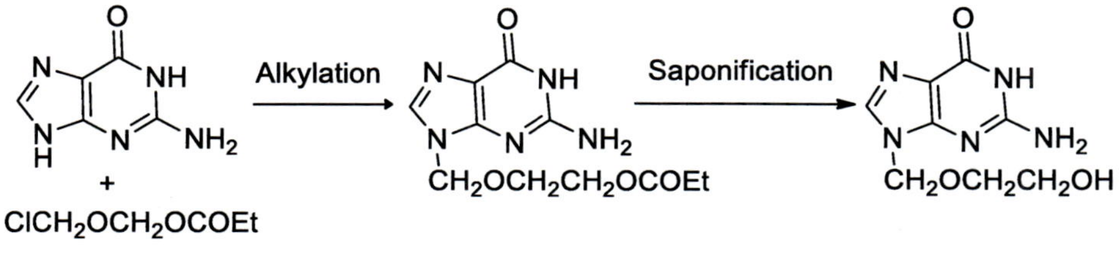

Retrosynthetic Analysis 2

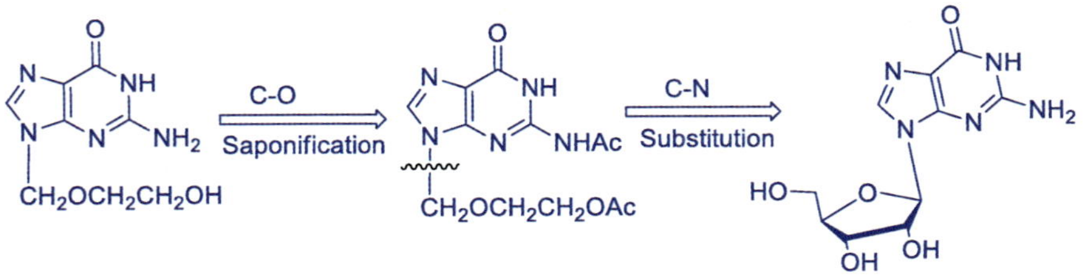

Chemical Synthesis 2

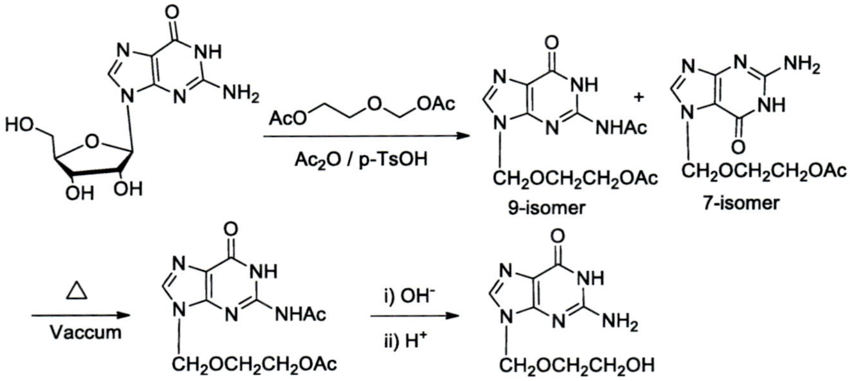

Retrosynthetic Analysis 3

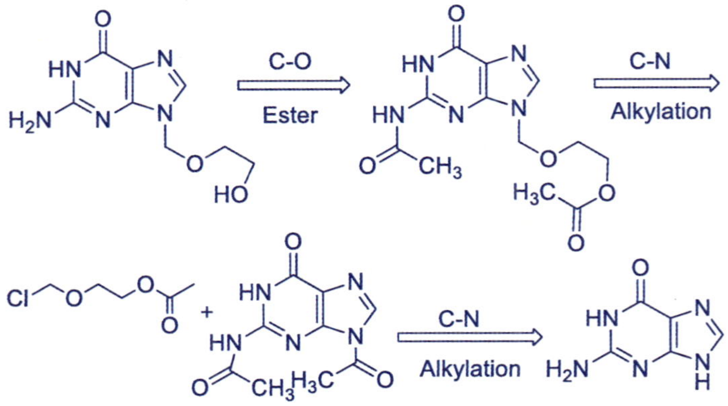

Chemical Synthesis 3:

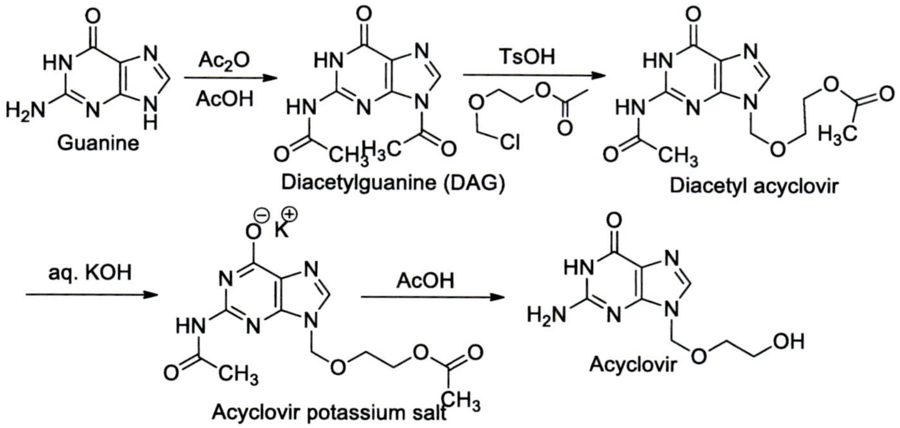

Phenobarbital

Retrosynthetic Analysis 1

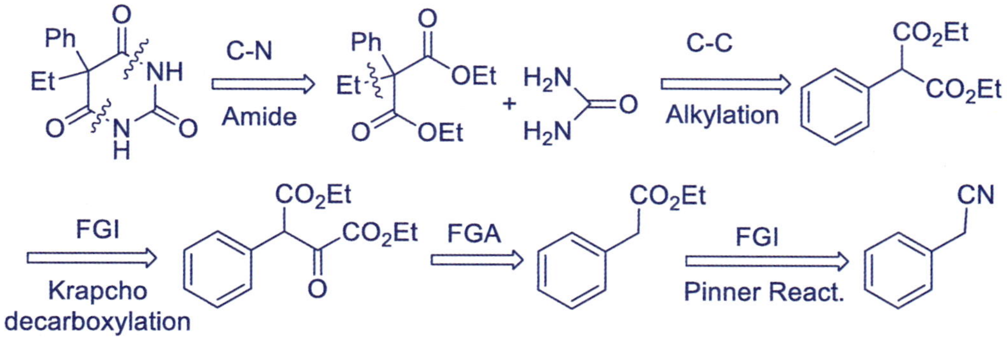

An alternative approaches is equally feasible and considered as most feasible pathway.

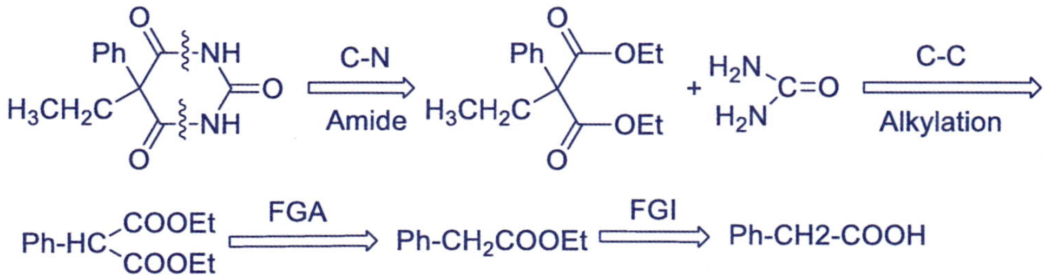

Chemical Synthesis 1

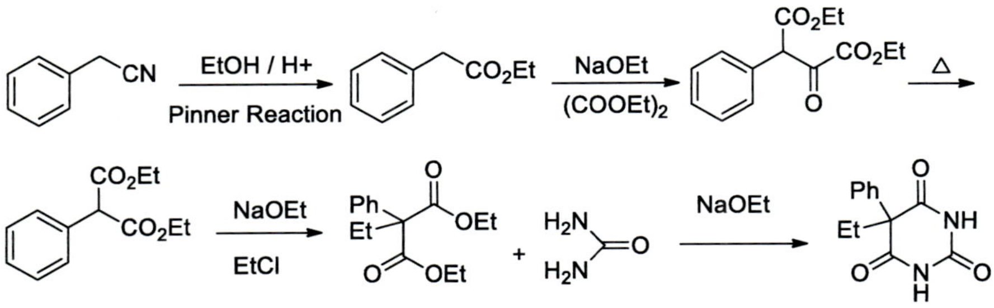

Retrosynthetic Analysis 2

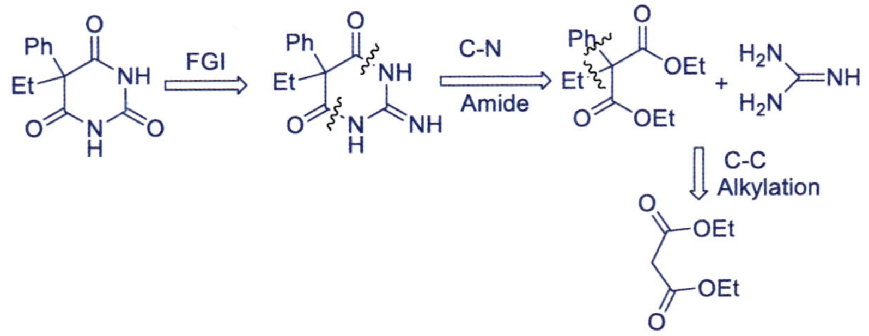

Chemical Synthesis 2

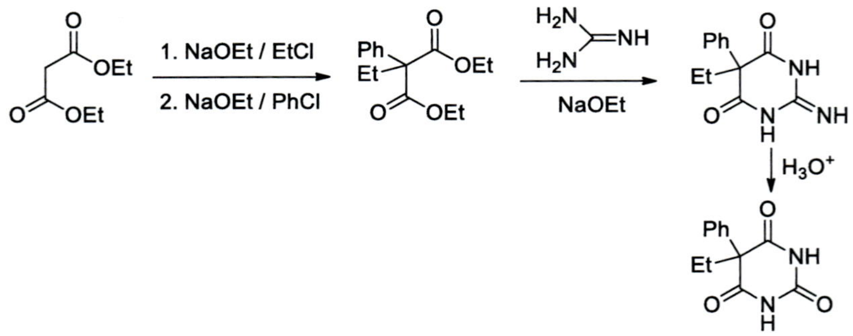

Diazepam

Retrosynthetic Analysis 1

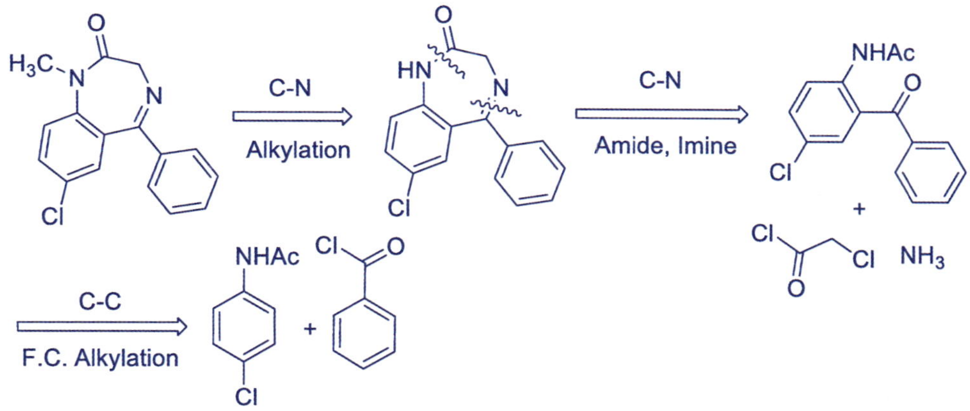

Chemical Synthesis 1

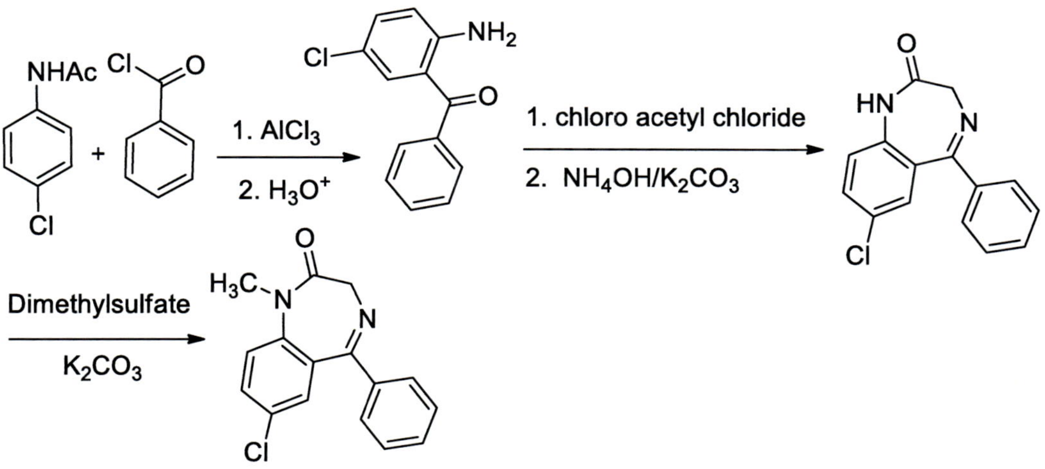

Retrosynthetic Analysis 2

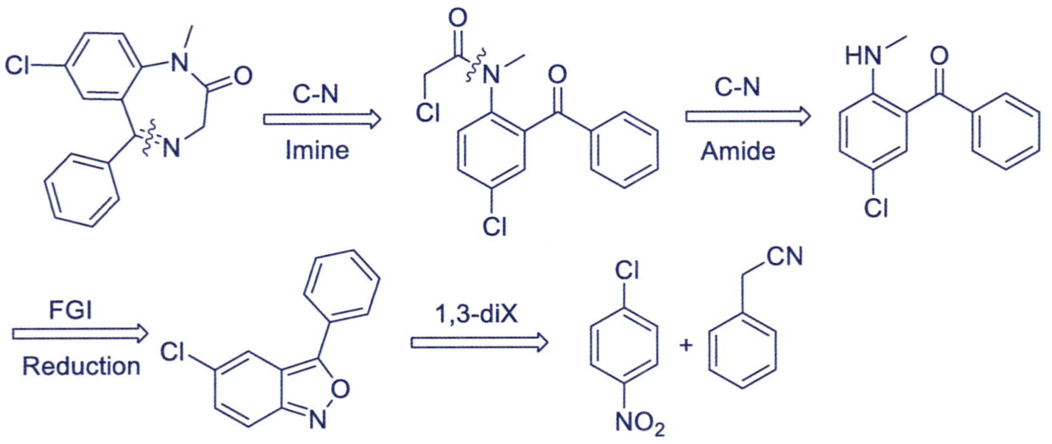

Chemical Synthesis 2

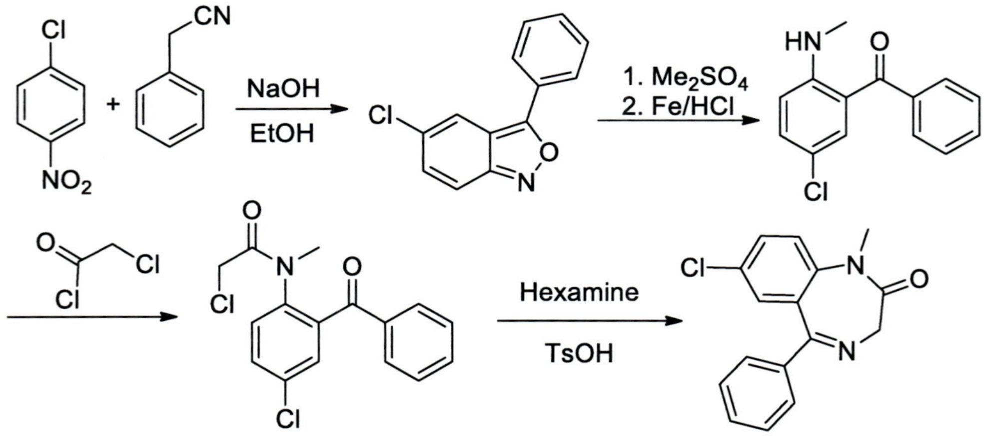

Retrosynthetic Analysis 3

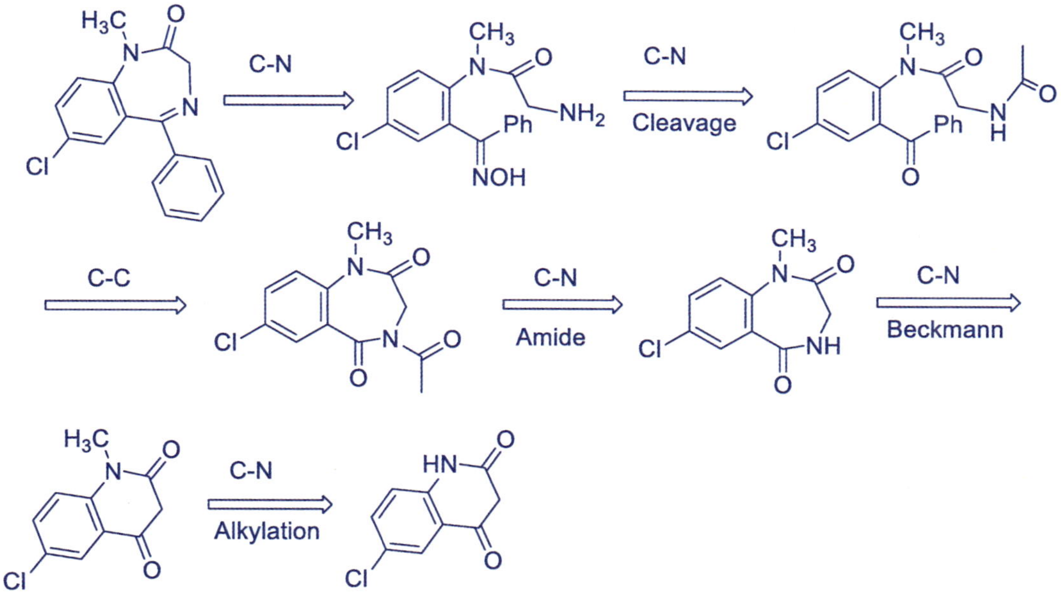

Chemical Synthesis 3

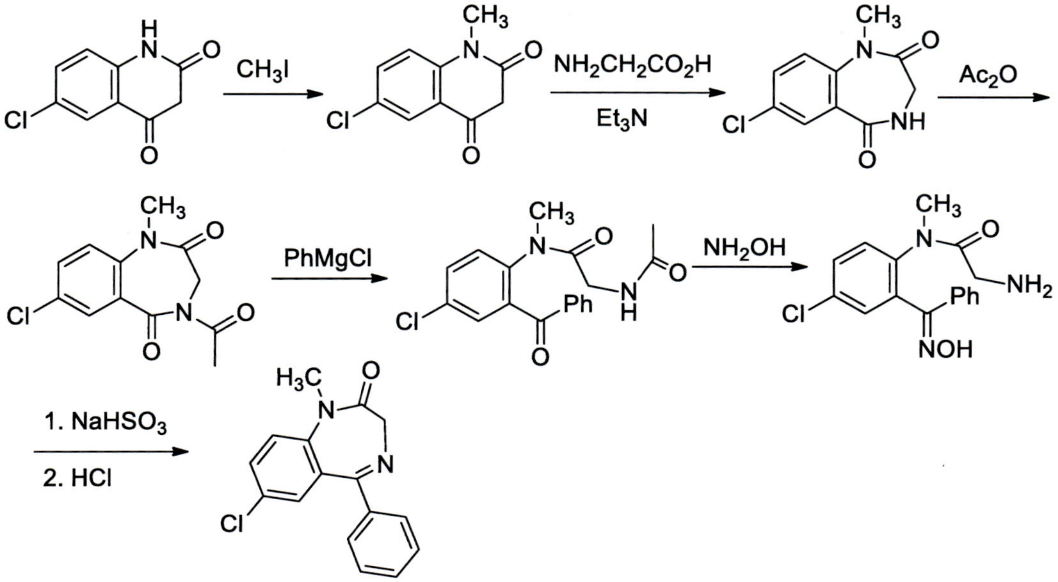

Glyceryl Trinitrate

Retrosynthetic Analysis 1

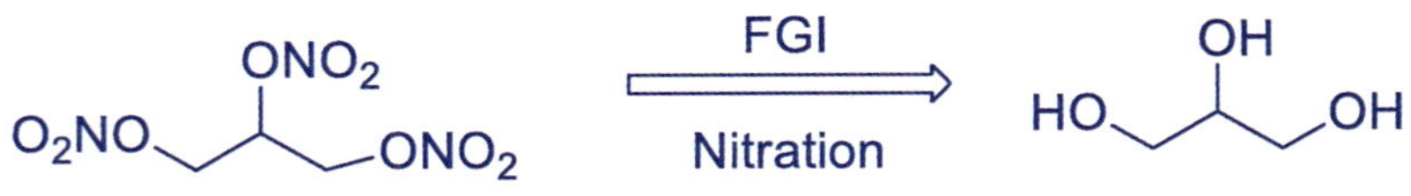

Chemical Synthesis 1

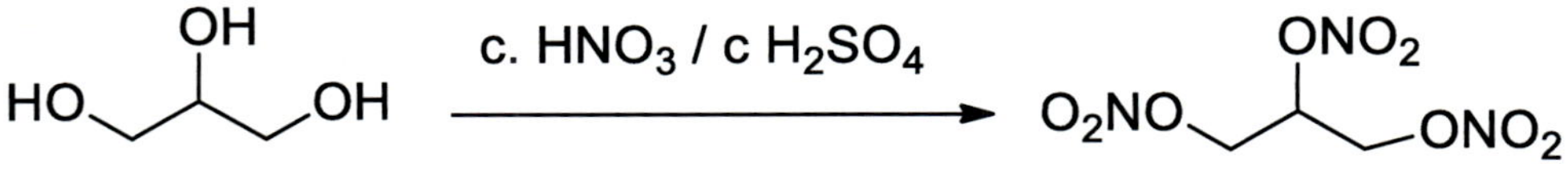

AZT- Zidovudine

Retrosynthetic Analysis 1

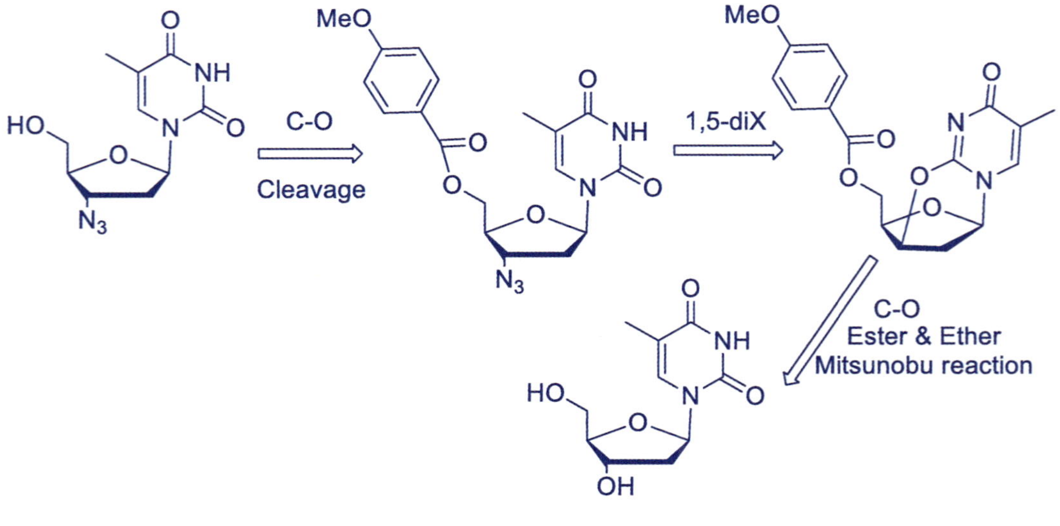

Chemical Synthesis 1

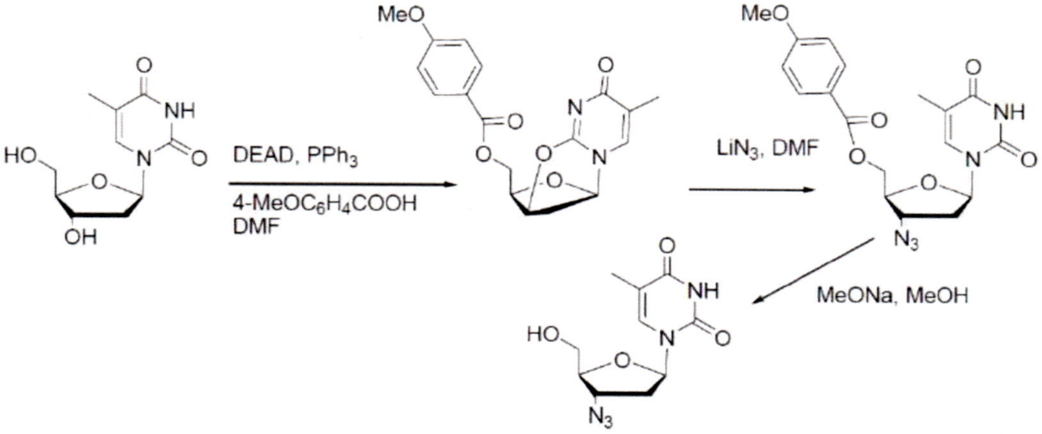

Retrosynthetic Analysis 2

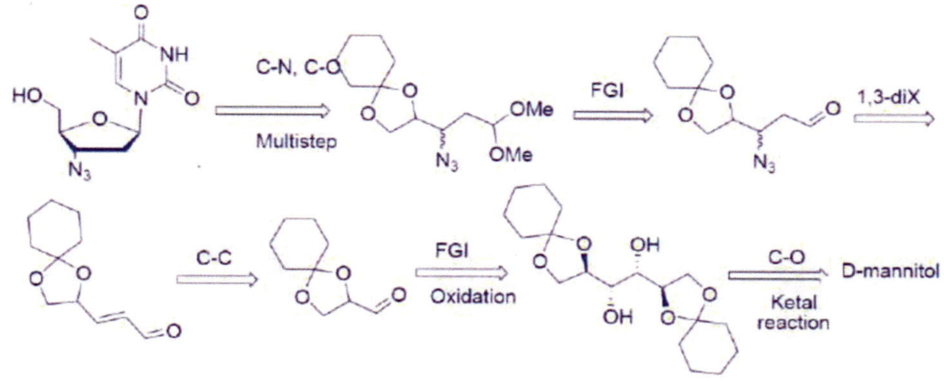

Chemical Synthesis 2

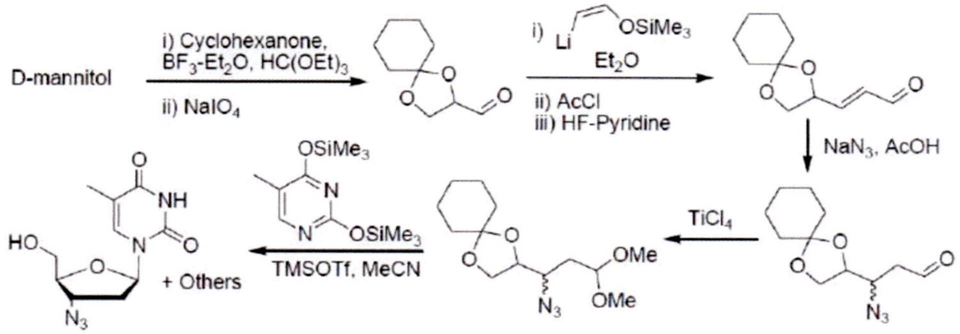

Retrosynthetic Analysis 3

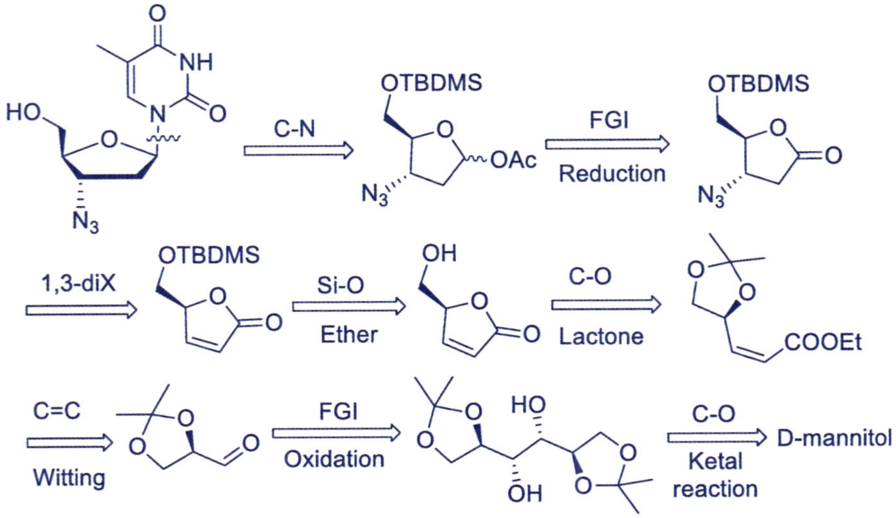

Chemical Synthesis 3

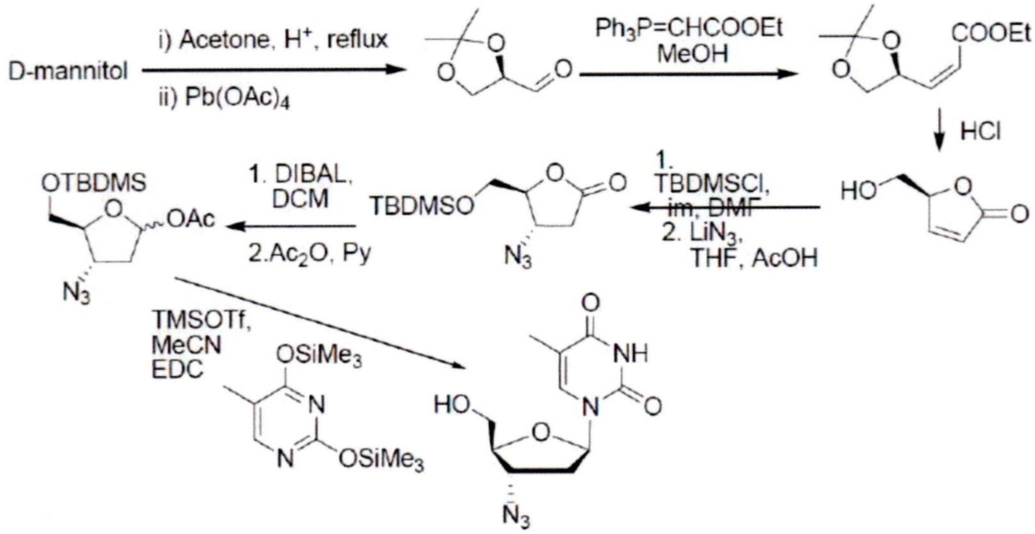

CHAPTER 6

Fermentation: Introduction

Abstract: This chapter explain aerobic and anaerobic fermentation and the path of fermentation in the cellular pathway. Few technologies *e.g.* DNA recombinant technology and polymerase chain reaction have been discussed in the very preliminary level in order to generate basic concept with the beginners.

Keywords: Drug discovery, Pharmaceuticals, Pharmaceutical chemistry, Pharmacology, Pharmacokinetics.

AEROBIC AND ANAEROBIC FERMENTATION

Fermentation is a cellular path of respiration, which occurs in the absence of oxygen. Thereby, it is more precisely called anaerobic respiration rather than aerobic fermentation (Table **1**). The two mechanisms of anaerobic fermentation are ethanol fermentation and lactic acid fermentation [35-37].

In anaerobic conditions, pyruvic acid is transformed by the organism into different pathways: *lactic acid fermentation*, *alcohol fermentation*, or *cellular (anaerobic) respiration*. Humans cannot ferment alcohol in their bodies as they lack the genetic information needed to do so.

Table 1. Aerobic and anaerobic fermentation.

Particulars	Aerobic Fermentation	Anaerobic Fermentation
Definition	Set of chemical reactions involved in the production of energy by completely oxidizing food	Chemical breakdown of organic substrates into ethanol or lactic acid by microorganisms in the absence of oxygen
Occurrence	cytoplasm and mitochondria	cytoplasm
Organisms	higher animals and plants	yeast, parasites, and bacteria
Oxygen	Uses molecular oxygen as the final electron acceptor in the electron transport chain	Does not use oxygen

Samir Kumar Mandal and Rebeca Ghanta

Water	Produces six water molecules per glucose molecule	Does not produce water
Substrate Oxidization	Glucose is completely broken down into carbon dioxide and oxygen	Glucose is incompletely oxidized either into ethanol and lactic acid
NAD+ Regeneration	NAD^+ regeneration occurs in the electron transport chain	NAD^+ regeneration occurs during the partial oxidation of pyruvate
ATP Production	ATP is a yield during the NAD^+ regeneration	ATP is not a yield during the NAD^+ regeneration
Efficiency (ATPs)	Produces 36 ATPs	Produces 2 ATPs
Toxicity	Aerobic respiration is non-toxic to the organism	Lactic acid, which is produced during the lactic acid fermentation, is toxic to tissues

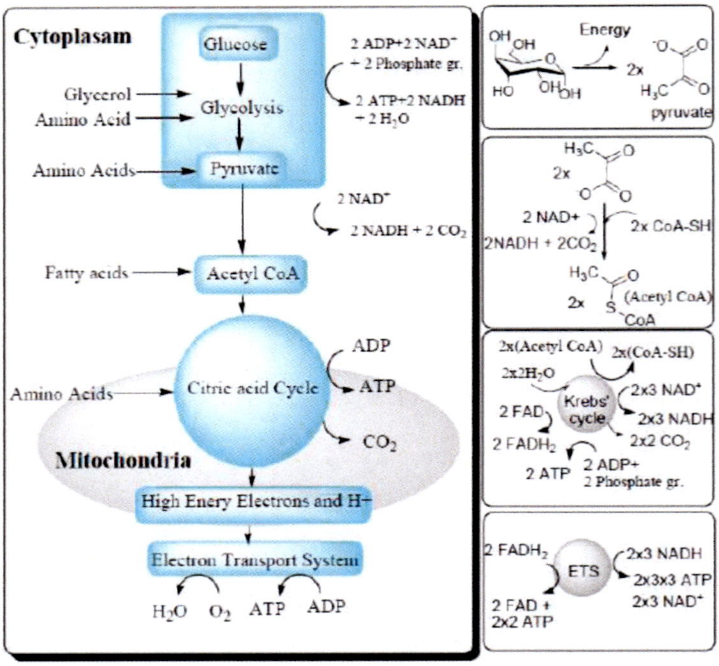

Fig. (1). ATP production path.

Alcohol fermentation is the formation of alcohol from sugar. In the glycolysis pathways under anaerobic conditions, yeast converts glucose to pyruvic acid, then goes one step farther, converting pyruvic acid into ethanol. The ability of different organisms in fermentation varies. They ferment pyruvic acid into other chemicals, such as lactic acid. Humans ferment lactic acid in muscles where oxygen is insufficient, a case of localized anaerobic conditions. This lactic acid causes muscle stiffness and feels like a lazy person (couch-potato). The stiffness goes away after a few days since the lactic acid is converted into ATP *via* the normal aerobic respiration pathways (Fig. **1**) [38].

When oxygen is present (aerobic conditions), most organisms will undergo two more steps, **Kreb's Cycle** and Electron Transport, to produce their ATP. In eukaryotes, these processes occur in the mitochondria, while in prokaryotes, they occur in the cytoplasm.

Aerobic Respiration

A set of chemical reactions is involved in the production of energy by completely oxidizing food in the presence of oxygen [35, 39]. This occurs in higher animals and plants. The first step of aerobic respiration is Glycolysis, which occurs in the cytoplasm of all cells independently without oxygen. This is also the first step of glucose degradation in anaerobic respiration. During Glycolysis, glucose is broken down into two pyruvate molecules, generating 2ATPs. In this step, two molecules of NADH are also formed by obtaining electrons from glyceraldehydes-3--phosphate. The pyruvate is entered into the mitochondria to form acetyl-CoA from pyruvate with the elimination of two molecules of carbon dioxide *via* oxidative decarboxylation of pyruvate. Acetyl-CoA then enters into the **Krebs cycle**, citric acid cycle.

In this cycle, a single glucose molecule is completely oxidized into six carbon dioxides (1x2 from pyruvate to acetylCoA + 2x2 in TCA cycle) molecules, generating 2GTPs, 6NADH and $2FADH_2$. NADH and $FADH_2$ are combined with oxygen to generate ATP during oxidative phosphorylation. This occurs in the inner membrane of mitochondria *via* transferring electrons through a series of carriers in the **E**lectron **T**ransport **C**hain (**ETC**). The total yield of aerobic respiration is 36 ATPs (Fig. **2**) [37].

$$\mathbf{C_6H_{12}O_6 + 6O_2 \longrightarrow 6H_2O + 6CO_2 + 2900\ KJ/mol}$$

In this cycle, a single glucose molecule is completely oxidized into **$6CO_2$** = (1x2 from pyruvate to acetylCoA + 2x2 in TCA cycle) molecules
And
2GTPs= (2x1in TCA cycle)
And
6NADH= (2x3in TCA cycle)
And
$2FADH_2$. =(2x1in TCA cycle)

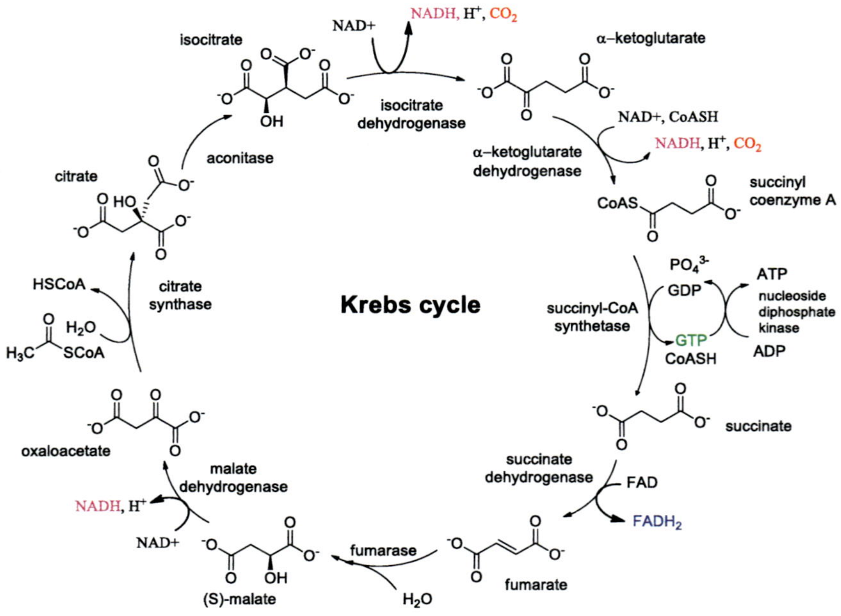

The total yield of ATPs in aerobic respiration is 36-38 ATPs from a single glucose molecule .
8 ATPs **= 2ATPs +2NADH** (1x2 ATPs + 2x3 ATPs) from glucose to pyruvate
And
6 ATPs **= 2NADH** (2x3 ATPs) from pyruvate to actyl CoA
And
18 ATPs = **6NADH** = (6x3 ATPs) from TCA cycle
And
2 ATPs **= 2ATPs** from TCA cycle [succinate to succinyl Coenzyme A]
And
4 ATPs **= 2FADH2** =(2xATPs) from TCA cycle

---

38 ATPs = [2ATPs+2NADH] + [2NADH] + [6NADH + 2FADH2 + 2ATPs]

ETS = Oxidation of NADH produces 3ATPs
Oxidation of FADHw2 produces 2 ATPs

Fig. (2). Krebs cycle.

Anaerobic Respiration

A set of chemical reactions is involved in the absence of oxygen to break down food into simple organic compounds, generating energy in the form of ATP [35,

-37]. This occurs in the cytoplasm of microorganisms like some bacteria, Yeast, and parasitic worms to produce only 2 ATPs.

Two categories of anaerobic respiration are identified. The first one of anaerobic respiration takes place through Glycolysis and then incomplete oxidation of pyruvate either into lactic acid or ethanol. The process is called fermentation. The resulting pyruvate is converted into ethanol in Yeast and some bacteria. In plants, when oxygen is absent, ethanol is produced by anaerobic respiration.

The final electron acceptor and the hydrogen acceptor are the simple organic end products. The end products are secreted into the medium as waste metabolites.

Ethanol Fermentation

$$\mathbf{C_6H_{12}O_6 \longrightarrow 2C_2H_5OH + 2CO_2 + 118\ KJ/mol}$$

Lactic Acid Fermentation

$$\mathbf{C_6H_{12}O_6 \longrightarrow 2C_3H_6O_3 + 120\ KJ/mol}$$

TECHNOLOGY BASED COMMERCIALIZATION OF FERMENTATION

With the need for amino acids, vitamins (primary metabolite), antibiotics (secondary metabolite), and industrial enzymes, commercial synthesis took a large area to balance the supply line, but fermented production is crucial with ecological significance [35-37].

Primary Metabolites

Primary metabolites are microbial products made during the exponential growth phase whose synthesis is an integral part of the normal growth process.

Secondary Metabolites

Secondary metabolites are microbial products that have a major effect on the health, nutrition and economics of our society.

With the development of the **DNA recombinant technology**, many approaches have been come into play to increase the efficiency of their biosynthesis [35d]. This allows the fulfillment of the aim to increases production along with new final product development by manipulating the pathways to direct the biosynthetic fluxes in one particular direction. This rather reduces the purification of unambiguous by product.

DNA Recombinant Technology [35]

It is the joining together of **DNA** molecules from two different species [5, 36, 37]. Recombinant DNA is inserted into a host organism to produce new genetic combinations that are of value to science, medicine, agriculture, and industry.

Steps: Recombinant DNA is a synthetic DNA which contains segments from more than one source. Preparation of recombinant DNA needs three key elements:

- A plasmid DNA in which a new DNA segment will be inserted.
- A restriction endonuclease, an enzyme that cleaves the DNA at specific site.
- Another DNA segment that will be inserted into plasmid DNA.

Preparation of recombinant DNA started with the cleavage of plasmid DNA in the presence of restriction endonuclease, which can recognize a specific sequence of bases in a DNA and cut the DNA at a particular position. As a result, two ends with unpaired bases of linear double-stranded DNA produced as plasmid DNA are circular and double-stranded. A second DNA is cut with the same restriction endonuclease and results in two sticky ends that are complementary to those of the plasmid DNA. Now, these strands are combined in the presence of DNA ligase enzyme to form recombinant DNA, which is larger than plasmid DNA (Fig. **3**).

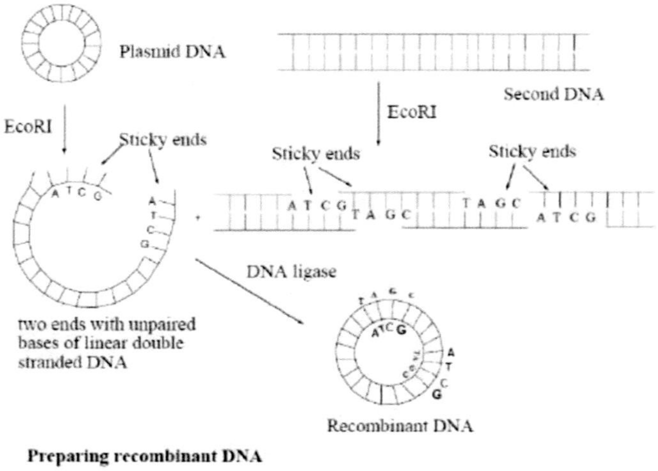

Fig. (3). Preparing recombinant DNA.

This technology helps find the crucial proteins required for health problems and dietary purposes safely, affordably, and sufficiently.

Techniques of recombinant DNA technology, gene therapy, and genetic modifications are also widely used for the purpose of bioremediation and treating serious diseases.

Applications of DNA Recombinant Technology [5]

(a) Therapeutic products

- Vaccines
- Antibodies
- Recombinant proteins
- Anti-cancer drugs

(b) Genetically modified products

- Genetically modified crops
- Genetically modified microbes
- Genetically modified vegetables

(c) Diagnosis

- Gene therapy
- Monitoring devices
- Therapeutic strategies

(d) Energy applications

- Bioethanol
- Biomethanol
- Biohydrogen

Polymerase Chain Reaction

Polymerase chain reaction (PCR) amplifies a specific portion of a DNA molecule [5, 7, 36, 37]. The requirements for PCR are:

- Segment of DNA
- Two primers
- DNA polymerase enzyme
- Nucleoside triphosphates

Each cycle of polymerase chain reaction involves three steps:

Step I: Unwinding the double-strand into a single strand by heating.

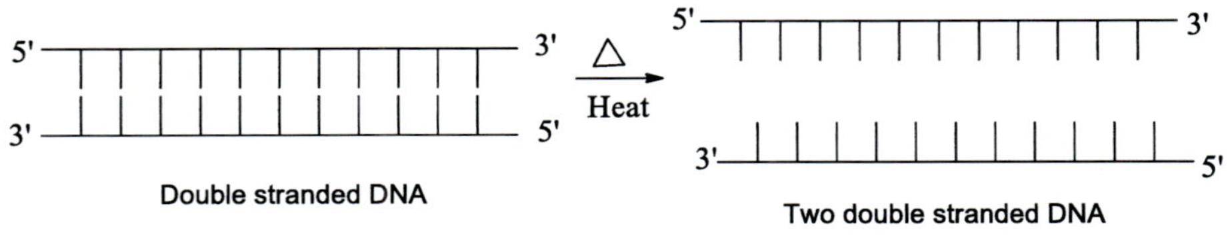

Step II: Addition of primers that are complementary to either end of the DNA segment to be amplified.

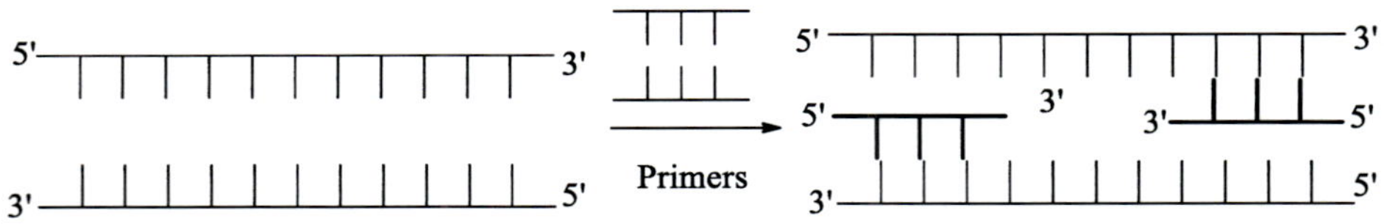

Primers add to the single-stranded DNA by H-bond and form a short double-stranded DNA segment. New nucleotides will add to the 3′end of the primer.

Step III: Addition of nucleotides to lengthen the DNA segment.

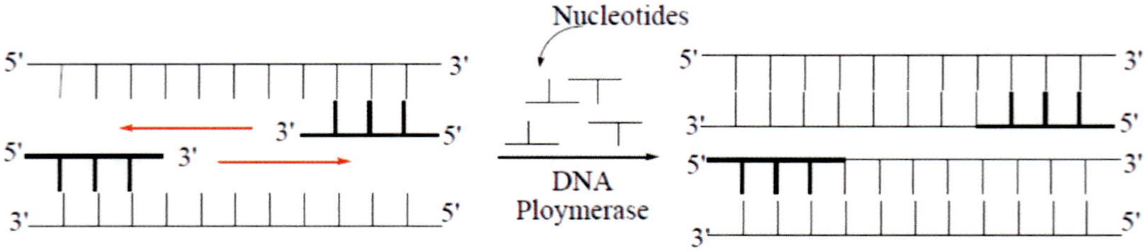

DNA polymerase catalyzed the addition of new nucleotides to the 3′ end of the primer and extended the chain of the new strand, which is complementary to the existing strand. Therefore, two DNA molecules are produced from one DNA molecule and multiplication of DNA can be done by PCR technology.

In wine production, Polymerase Chain Reaction (PCR)-Denaturing Gradient Gel Electrophoresis (DGGE) helps to identify the Lactic Acid Bacteria (LAB) contaminants. This is particularly based on the PCR amplification of a DNA fragment from the region V1 of 16S rDNA gene followed by a DGGE technique. The main contaminant is *Lactobacillus* spp and *Pediococcus* spp.

CHAPTER 7

Production of Commodities

Abstract: Synthesis of commercials like ethanol and citric acid have been discussed via 'Low-Value, High-Volume' production criteria via fermentation process. Feedstock, micro-organism, media and condition of fermentation processes discussed here.

Keywords: Drug discovery, Pharmaceuticals, Pharmaceutical chemistry, Pharmacology pharmacokinetics.

INTRODUCTION

There are many useful commodities that are collected from fermentation [36, 38 -40]. From bread to beer, vinegar, yoghurt, cheese, and wine are well known fermented products that are used as daily essentials. Some other fermented products like xanthan gum (used in the ice-cream industry to prevent foam, paint industry for sticking to the brush but spreading smoothly from the brush to the surface) are also growing rapidly. With the development of biotechnology, the industry is critically dependent on the microbial fermentation process with the fulfillment of the commercial term "*low-value, high-volume product*" [35d].

Criteria of the Low-Value, High-Volume Product

- Completion of fermentation in a relatively short time
- Production of the desired product in relatively pure form

To fulfill these, the cost of nutrients (carbon, nitrogen, sulfur, phosphorus, vitamins, and minerals) and utilities (heating, cooling, air, *etc.*) and improved stains (microorganisms or other cells under the microscope) are very crucial. As the costs of nutrients are fluctuating at an alarming rate, flexibilities of nutrients choice are important. Genetic engineering is relentlessly developing stains to improve the microbial process, which is another important factor.

Microorganisms and fermentation media are very important for the high yield of the product. The basis for selecting fermentation microorganism are as follows:

- The strain that gives a high yield of the product should be selected.

Samir Kumar Mandal and Rebeca Ghanta (Eds.)

- The strain that grows rapidly with a high tolerance of a high concentration of sugar should be selected.
- The microorganism should have genetic stability.

The fermentation medium provides a substrate for product synthesis in a fermentor. The major and minor components in a fermentation media are as follows:.

- Major components:carbon and nitrogen source.
- Minor components: inorganic salts, vitamins, growth factors, anti-foaming agents, buffers, dissolved oxygen other dissolved gases, growth inhibitors, and enzymes.

Both Ethyl alcohol and citric acid are produced in anaerobic fermentation. Scientist Louis Pasteur (1860) showed that alcoholic fermentation is a part of yeast cells (higher fungi). Later, Buchner proved that this fermentation in yeast is due to an enzyme which catalyzed the conversion of sugar unit into alcohol. The three main phases of fermentation are preparation and inoculation, fermentation, and recovery.

Ingredients of Crude Media

The ingredients of crude media are given in Table **1**.

Inorganic Nutrients	Cations like magnesium ions, zinc ion and anions like nitrate, phosphates, sulphates, *etc.*
Carbon Source	Carbohydrates, such as glucose, fructose, mannitol, sorbitol, starch, cellulose including organic acids, fatty acids, proteins, peptides from different sources like Blackstrap molasses, Corn molasses, Beet molasses, sulphite waste liquor, Hydrol, Cannery waste, Corn, Rice, Rye, Milo, wheat potatoes, corn cobs, straws, wood waste, saw meal.
Nitrogen Source	Different salts of urea, ammonia, and nitrate. For non-proteolytic organisms, urea, ammonia and nitrate are used, while for proteolytic organisms Casein, Cereal grains, peptones, yeast extract, hydrolysate, and soybean meal are used.
Growth Factors	Yeast extract and beef extract
Buffers	On many occasions, media components such as protein, peptides, amino-acids act as good buffers at neutral pH. Inorganic buffers like K_2HPO_4, KH_2PO_4, and $CaCO_3$, *etc.*, can be added as and when required.

ETHYL ALCOHOL

Ethanol is the key ingredient of beverages, renewable fuels, universal solvents,and an important building block for higher member organics, including surface disinfectants and antiseptics. Alcoholic beverages are being used from old days to today but with the advancement of microbiology [41]. They are commonly called wine, beer, and whisky, and have an alcohol content of 10-12%, 8-10%, and 40-50%, respectively. Wine is commonly prepared from grapes but it may also be prepared from other fruits. On the other hand, beer is produced mainly from malted barley and wheat, while whiskey is produced from a variety of malted grains like barley, rye, maize, and wheat [36, 38].

Ethanol is produced by biological processes from sugars, such as glucose, fructose, sucrose, *etc.*, and bacteria, as well as fungi, are used as microbes [41]. The sugar is converted into alcohol and carbon dioxide under anaerobic conditions. For low-cost production, renewable feedstock that contains saccharides, starchy and cellulosic materials are used for this purpose. Other than fermentation, the petrochemical process is also useful for the production of ethanol.

Substrates	
Cellulosic material	*Candida* species for sulphite waste from the paper industry
Starchy materials	*Saccharomyces* species for starch like corn starch, potato starch, and wheat flour
Saccharides	*Saccharomyces* species for sugar cane molasses, beet molasses, hydrol, fruit juices
Diary waste	*Candida* species for dairy waste
Microorganisms	
Species of *Saccharomyces*	*Saccharomyces cerevisiae or Saccharomyces ellipsoideus*
Species of *Candida*	*Candida pseudotropicalis, Candida utilis*

The production of ethyl alcohol mostly depends on molasses in our country. For many purposes, for low-cost production, agricultural waste is pre-treated for removal of unwanted, toxic products and then converted into sugar form such that sugar can be easily utilized by the inoculum. Molasses is then diluted with water to a 10% sugar solution, called "**mash**" (process of combining a mix of grains) for fermentation. A yeast culture is added for inoculation of the media. The solution is made acidic (pH 4.0-5.0) by adding sulphuric acid to prevent the growth of unwanted bacteria. For active fermentation, ammonium sulphate and ammonium phosphates are continuously supplied in a concentration of about 0.015% for the nutrition of yeast. The temperature is maintained at 22-25 °C. The nutrient media is facilitated with a high amount of aeration and agitation for faster growth. Within a few hours, carbon dioxide gas is evolved and after a day, it appears to boil due to frothing. In this process, invertase enzyme hydrolyses sucrose (glycosidic linkage is α for glucose and β for fructose) into glucose and fructose. Glucose and fructose are then converted into ethyl alcohol and carbon dioxide by the enzyme zymase. Fermentation is completed within 2-3 days. The fermented liquor contains 6-8% alcohol, which is concentrated by fractional distillation by using an analyzer and rectifier column.

Biotin is one of the important growth factors in this fermentation. For this reason, beet molasses is also added to the medium.

$$C_{12}H_{22}O_{11} + H_2O \xrightarrow{\text{Invertage}} \underset{\text{glucose}}{C_6H_{12}O_6} + \underset{\text{fructose}}{C_6H_{12}O_6}$$

$$C_6H_{12}O_6 \xrightarrow{\text{Zymase}} 2\,C_2H_5OH + 2\,CO_2$$

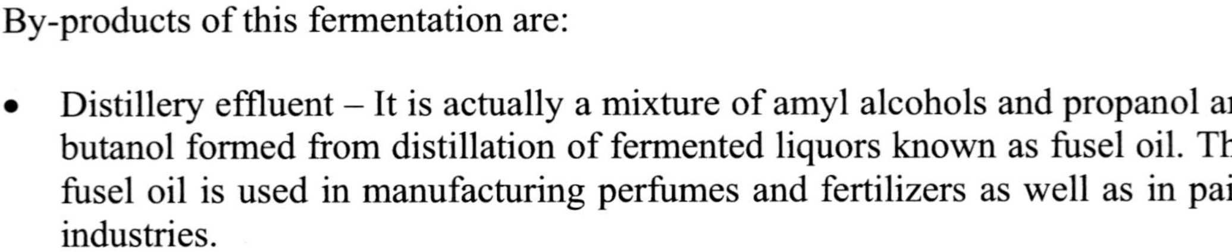

By-products of this fermentation are:

- Distillery effluent – It is actually a mixture of amyl alcohols and propanol and butanol formed from distillation of fermented liquors known as fusel oil. This fusel oil is used in manufacturing perfumes and fertilizers as well as in paint industries.
- The residual yeast cells are used in food material preparation.
- The carbon dioxide produced is purified and used as dry ice or used in carbonated drinks.

Fermentation

Wine (From Grapes)

The fermentation of grapes is used for the preparation of wine [35d, 36, 39]. The name of different wines is based on the type of grapes and source of production. There are five steps for making wine – harvesting, crushing and pressing (must formation), fermentation, clarification, and aging and bottling. The ripe grapes are collected on sunny days. Grapes are mashed or crushed and squeezed for juice along with skin and seeds, which are called "**must**". The cultured yeasts (pure and one strain in a dried or inactive state), commonly used *Saccharomyces cerevisiae species*, are added to allow alcoholic fermentation. The inactive state is activated by mixing with warm water or diluted grape juice. The yeast cells feed on the sugar in the **must** and there occurs conversion of sugar into alcohol and carbon dioxide. The temperature is maintained at 22-25 °C to get the best results. Alcohol, thus, produced in this method is half a gram for one gram of sugar. Therefore, for 10 % concentration of alcohol in the fermentation, the must should contain ≤20 % sugar for fermentation and this requires the addition of sugar into the must. At a specific point, sugar content of the must will stop decreasing. This indicates that boiling fermentation has stopped and is ready for separation. The duration of fermentation takes around 10-20days, depending on the final alcohol content in wine. For active fermentation, carbon (sugar), nitrogen, sulfur, phosphorus, and also nutrient sources, such as vitamins and minerals, are continuously supplied. Longer fermentation period causes a majority of sugar to turn into alcohol and this even kills the yeast, whereas shorter fermentation produces sweeter wine.

Beer (From Malted Cereal)

Fermentation of malted barley or wheat is used for the preparation of beer [35d, 36, 39]. The process of making beer is called brewing. This includes breaking a starch molecule into a sugar unit. The sugar solution obtained after brewing is called wort. Sugar in the wort is fermented by yeast into alcohol and carbon dioxide. Commonly used cultured yeasts are *Saccharomyces cerevisiae species.* For active fermentation, ammonium sulphate and ammonium phosphates are continuously supplied for the nutrition of yeast (***Escherichia coli*** **or** ***Saccharomyces cerevisiae***). The temperature is maintained at 22-25 °C. Within a few hours, carbon dioxide gas is evolved, and after a day, it appears to boil due to frothing. In this process, invertase enzyme hydrolyses sucrose. Fermentation is completed within 2-3 days. The fermented liquor contains 6-8% of alcohol, which is concentrated by fractional distillation.

The grains of wheat, rice, barley, and potatoes are milled in a mill and made into a slurry with water. The slurry is warmed to 65 °C and then heated to 180 °C for a minute. The starch solution is then treated with malt, and seeds of barly are germinated at 50 °C for half an hour. Now the enzyme diastase in malt hydrolyses starch (α-1, 4-glycosidic linkage in starch whereas β-1,4 glycosidic linkage in cellulose) into sugar maltose. The liquor is cooled to 15-20 °C and fermented with yeast. The maltase enzyme present in yeast hydrolyses maltose into glucose. Glucose is then converted into ethyl alcohol and carbon dioxide by the enzyme zymase. The fermented liquor contains 8-10% alcohol, which is concentrated by fractional distillation.

$$\underset{\text{starch}}{n(C_6H_{10}O_5)} + nH_2O \xrightarrow{\text{diastase}} \underset{\text{maltose}}{n\,C_{12}H_{22}O_{11}}$$

$$\underset{\text{maltose}}{C_{12}H_{22}O_{11}} \xrightarrow{\text{maltase}} \underset{\text{glucose}}{2\,C_6H_{12}O_6}$$

$$C_6H_{12}O_6 \xrightarrow{\text{Zymase}} 2\,C_2H_5OH + 2\,CO_2$$

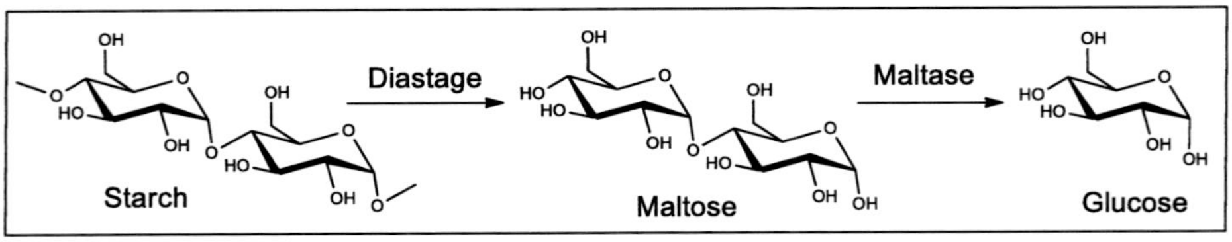

CITRIC ACID

Citric acid is an intermediate of the ubiquitous Krebs cycle (citric acid cycle), and therefore, it is present in every living organism [35d, 36, 39]. Citric acid is available in citrus fruits (lemon, oranges, *etc*). In 1784, Swedish chemist, Karl Wilhelm Scheele extracted citric acid from lemon juice and a few years later, this was adopted by England for commercial production of citric acid using lemons. After a long time, the economical industrial process was developed by James N. Curie in 1917. He discovered that the fermentation of glucose, sucrose, and molasses by mould *aspergillus niger* gave significant amounts of citric acid [42a]. Since then, Pfizer started the commercial production of citric acid. This is used in carbonated drinks, and approximately 70% of the total production of jams and jellies and other products like detergents, pharmaceuticals, cosmetics, toiletries, *etc.* One of the main uses of citric acid is as potassium citrate in the medicinal field, where potassium citrate works within the urinary bladder and increases the urinary pH and urine citrate levels. Citrate inhibits stone formation by complexing with calcium in the urine. Potassium citrate helps by inhibiting the crystallization of stone-forming salts such as calcium oxalate, calcium phosphate, and uric acid. Industrially, citric acid is largely used in metal finishing and cleaning, followed by lubricants, chelating agents, animal feeds, and plasticizers.

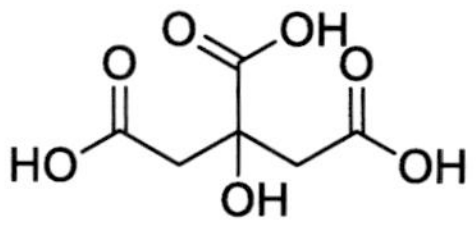

citric acid

Citric acid is a primary metabolic product formed in the tricarboxylic acid (Krebs) cycle [6]. Glucose is the predominant carbon source for citric acid production. The biosynthetic pathway for citric acid production involves glycolysis, wherein glucose is converted into two molecules of pyruvate. Pyruvate is transformed into acetyl CoA in mitochondria and condensed with oxaloacetate in the presence of citrate synthase to give citrate (Fig. **1**).

With the demand of growing markets, this is important to discover and develop better production techniques to improve production yields. In large-scale production, it is necessary and important to develop a production process to be environmentally friendly by utilizing readily available and inexpensive agro-industrial waste products with high yields [38].

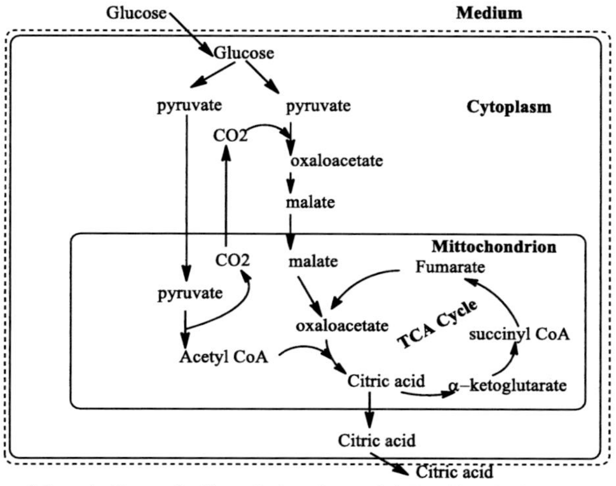

Fig. (1). Schematic diagram for biosynthetic pathway of citric acid production.

Fermentation is one such process. microbial conversion has been adapted in industries using *Aspergillus niger* from organic materials to citric acid under specific conditions. Yeasts are capable of producing citric acid from *n*-alkanes and carbohydrates, but it produces large quantities of isocitric acid (Fig. **2**). Fermentation is advantageous due to its operational simplicity, easiest systems, and less energy consumption with lower technical skill.

Substrates	
Hydrocarbons	*n*-paraffin, glycerol, olive oil, rapeseed oil, palm oil, and soya bean oil.
Starchy materials	Corn starch, hydrolysate starch, yam bean starch, wood hemicellulose
Molasses	Beet molasses, blackstrap molasses, cane molasses
Microorganisms	
Species of *Aspergillus*	*A. Niger, A. wenti, A. foetidus, A. aculeatus, A. awamori, A. fonsecaeus, A. phoenicis* and *A. carbonaries, Trichoderma viride, Mucor pyriformis etc*
Species of Yeast	*Candida tropiclaus, Candida oleophilis, Candida guilermondi, Yarrowia lipolytica, Torulopsis, Hansenula, Debaromyces, Torula, Pichia, Kloekera, Saccharomyces, Zygosaccharomyces, etc.*

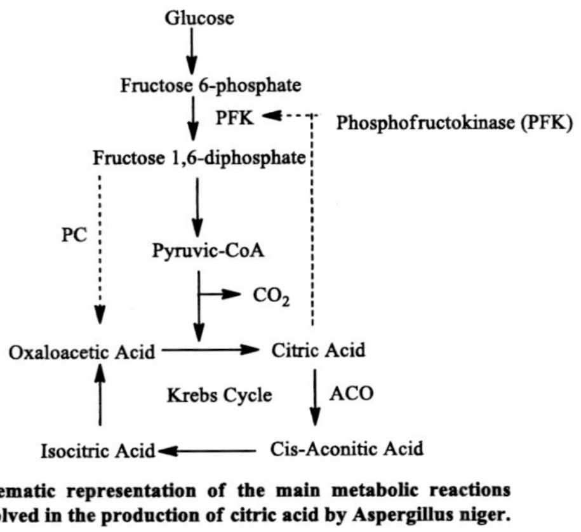

Fig. (2). Shematic representation of the main metabolic reactions involved in the production of citric acid by *Aspergillus niger.*

Factors Affecting Fermentation

There are several factors that affect the fermentation process, which are as follows [38]:

- **Concentration and Type of Carbon Source**: Monosaccharides and disaccharides are the ideal carbon sources as they are more rapidly metabolized by the fungus than polysaccharides. This helps better yields. Sucrose is superior to glucose, fructose, and lactose due to the strong extracellular mycelium-bound invertase of *A. niger*, which rapidly hydrolyses sucrose at low pH. But large scale production of pure monosaccharides and disaccharides is beyond the economical standard. Therefore, wastes from sugar refineries, for example, cane and beet molasses, are used for this purpose but after pretreatment. The concentration of carbon source is also important and the experiment suggests that the maximum concentration is 14-22%.

- **The pH of the Fermentation Medium**: The pH (usually <3) of the fermentation medium plays a major role during the sporulation and production phase. During fermentation, different acids, such as citric acid and the unwanted gluconic and oxalic acid, are produced. But the metabolic activity of the microbes can control the pH by different means. Some of the microbes can reduce the pH (*Aspergillus*, *Rhizopus* and *Penicillium* species are able to reduce the pH quickly to below 3) and some can be adjusted to a particular pH (*Sporotrichum* and *Pleurotus* species produce a more stable pH between 4 and 5).

- **Phosphate and Nitrogen Limitations**: Nitrogen sources *e.g.*, ammonium nitrate, ammonium sulphate, peptone, malt extract, urea, are important as they are a part of a cell's proteins and required for cellular metabolism. For this, ammonium salts, such as ammonium nitrate and ammonium sulphate, are used as supplements with later being preferred due to less accumulation of unwanted oxalic acid. A usual nitrogen salt that remains in the solution is 0.2-0.25 % (w/V) for better yield. Phosphorous source *e.g.*, potassium dihydrogen phosphate, is another factor for the same. Experiments suggest that phosphorus concentration of 0.5–5 g/l is required for fungal growth and, consequently, for good citric acid production.

- **Concentration of Alcohols**: The results suggest that the effect of alcohols has a profound positive effect on the formation of citric acid from different carbon sources. The optimum level of alcohol (methanol/ethanol /n-propanol / iso-propanol) lies between 1% and 3% for good production of citric acid.

- **Aeration**: Aeration rate is important for the fermentation of citric acid. Increased rate of aeration decreases the partial pressure of carbon dioxide and consequently results in better yields. High levels of carbon dioxide damage the final biomass and concentrations of citrate. Increased aeration rate evenly across the medium with similar intensity gives better yield.

- **The Concentrations of Trace Elements**: Though oxygen and sugar are required in excess, for nutrition, trace amounts of manganese, phosphate and nitrogen are required for the superior fermentation process. Beet molasses is superior to cane molasses since high content of trace metals, such as magnesium, zinc, manganese, calcium and iron, remainin cane molasses, which are all harmful in the synthesis of citric acid.

Fermentation

Production of citric acid is done from the purified and dilute molasses (10-20 % sugar solution). Molasses, remaining part after sugar extraction from the sugar syrup made from sugar cane, is treated with $K_4Fe(CN)_6$ at pH 4.5 and 90 °C for 15 min and then the precipitate is removed by filtration to make it suitable for fermentation. The solution is made 10% (w/v) for optimum yield. For active fermentation, ammonium nitrate or urea, potassium bisulfate, magnesium sulfates are continuously supplied for the nutrition of bacteria. The solution is made acidic (pH 3.0-4.5) by adding hydrochloric acid, and pH>4 accumulates oxalic acid. The temperature is maintained at 25-35 °C. The system is sterile with steam to prevent unwanted growth of microorganisms. Now, fermentation is carried out for almost 10 days with *aspergillus niger* when air bubbles through the solution. Thus, it becomes an aerobic reaction. The citric acid so produced is neutralized with a lime solution to precipitate as calcium citrate. The precipitate is filtered and decomposed to citric acid with a calculated amount of sulfuric acid. Calcium sulfate is separated and the filtrate is concentrated to get citric acid.

$$C_{12}H_{22}O_{11} + H_2O + 3O_2 \longrightarrow 2C_6H_8O_7 + 4H_2O$$

Industrial Process

In industrial manufacturing, the two main processes are - surface process and submerged process. Another fermentation process is solid-state fermentation or the Koji process. This process uses waste agro-product for the production of citric acid.

Surface Processes

Most of Asian countries use surface processes for the production of citric acid. Wheat bran or pulp from sweet potato starch is used as culture media [42b]. The ideal pH of the medium for this process is 4-5, which is adjusted before sterilization of the medium. After sterilization, the inoculum in the form of spores of *A. niger* is spread as layers, usually having a thickness of 3-6 cm and incubated at 28°C. For acceleration of the growth of the organisms, α-amylase is added. For maximal production of citric acid, the optimal period for this fermentation is about 80-100 hours. Once the process is over, citric acid is extracted into hot water and then isolated.

Submerged Processes

Submerged Process is considered the world's best process for the production of citric acid [42g]. This process is highly efficient and automated, one that requires advanced control technology with trained personnel. It is badly influenced by trace metals and other impurities. Commonly stirred tanks and aerated towers with high-quality stainless steel are used as bioreactors. In these bioreactors, air sparging is allowed from the base of the fermenter.The optimum supply of O_2 is 20-25% of saturation value for good production of citric acid, whereas the ideal aeration rate is in the range of 0.2-1 vvm (volume/volume/ minute). Forked and bulbous hyphae and branches like mycelium, part of a fungus or fungus-like bacterial colony, are responsible for the good yield of citric acid. Loose and filamentous mycelium, with limited branches, produces no citric acid at all. To prevent foam formation, anti-foaming agents like lard oil and mechanical anti-foaming devices are used for this process. For industrial production, the optimal condition is about 250-280 hours to obtain 100- 110 g/l of citric acid from 140 g/l of sucrose with biomass (dry weight) of 8-12 g/l.

Recovery

The culture broth is filtered and then mycelium is washed off. An unwanted by-product, oxalic acid, produced in the fermentation is removed by precipitation at pH< 3. Then, culture broth is adjusted to pH 7.2 and temperature 70-90 °C to precipitate out citric acid. For further purification of citric acid, it is dissolved in sulfuric acid to precipitate calcium sulfate and then treated with activated charcoal, cation and anion-exchangers and crystallization steps sequentially. To get citric acid monohydrate, it is crystallized below 36 °C but above 40 °C, citric acid is crystallized into an anhydrous form. Though citric acid monohydrate is the main commercial of citric acid, the degree of purity of citric acid thus produced depends on the purpose for which it is required. Usually, food grade citric acid is used in pure forms, but for industrial use, it can be used in a crude form.

CHAPTER 8

Production of Antibiotics

Abstract: In this chapter, brief discovery of certain antibiotics, their mode of action, their inactivity have been discussed in basic level. With the importance in present era, modern technologies at very preliminary level have discussed for the synthesis of some microbial product like Penicillin, Cephalosporin, Chloromycetin, Streptomycin *etc.* Their natural and commercial production process and development described in a simple way.

Keywords: Drug discovery, Pharmaceuticals, Pharmaceutical chemistry, Pharmacology, Pharmacokinetics.

INTRODUCTION

Antibiotics are chemical substances produced by microorganisms that kill or inhibit the growth of other microorganisms. The development of antibiotics, as agents, for the treatment of infectious diseases is more important in the practice of medicine [6, 43b, h]. Antibiotics are products of secondary metabolism that can be produced commercially by microbial fermentation. With the need for antibiotics, commercial synthesis took a large area to balance the supply line, but fermented production is crucial with ecological significance. Around 500 antibiotics were known in 1961, but currently, the number has reached beyond 8000.

With the development of DNA recombinant technology, there are many approaches that have come into play to increase the efficiency of antibiotic biosynthesis. This allows the fulfillment of the aim to increase the production along with new final product development. This requires manipulation of the pathways to direct the biosynthetic fluxes in one particular direction. Ultimately, in view of commercialization, it reduces the purification of the unambiguous by-product [35d].

PENICILLIN

The most famous example of an antibiotic is penicillin, which was observed by Alexander Fleming in 1929. He observed that the growth of *Staphylococcus aureus* was inhibited by a contaminant *Penicillium notatum* culture. The antibiotic produced by this fungus was named penicillin. Penicillin inhibited the growth and development of other microorganism and was used in the medicinal field, veterinary as well as the agricultural field [43a]. Benzylpenicillin (penicillin G, R=

Samir Kumar Mandal and Rebeca Ghanta

benzyl) was the first antibiotic produced at a large scale by submerged fermentation procedures in the early 1940s. Most of the penicillins are prepared *via* semi-synthetic approaches. The widely used semi-synthetic penicillin is ampicillin (R =D -α-aminobenzyl).

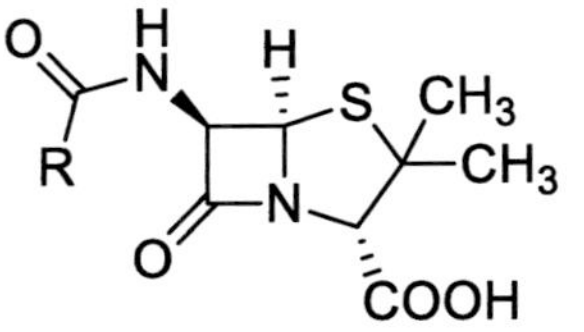

General structure of Penicillins

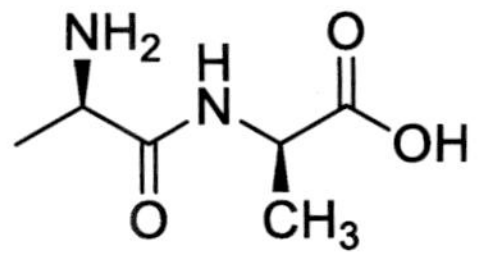

D-alanyl-D-alanine

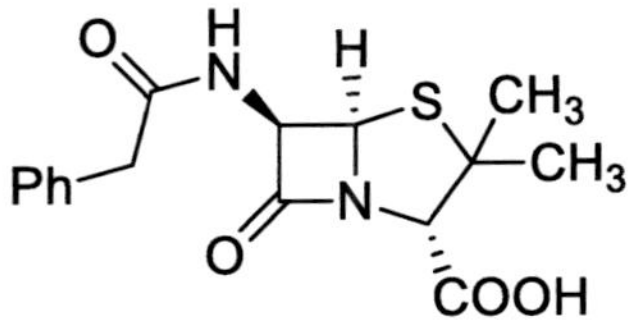

Penicillin G

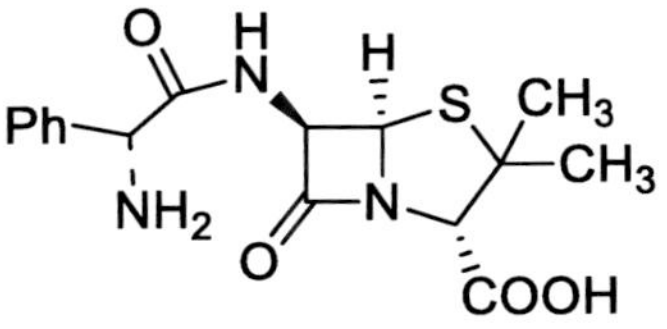

Ampicillin

Penicillins are used against both Gram-positive bacteria as well as Gram-negative bacteria. These are structural analogs of D-alanyl-D-alanine and bind to the active site of the transpeptidase. Lactam ring of this antibiotic gets attached to DD transpeptidase cell enzyme and inhibits the formation of cross-linkage in the cell wall. The transpeptidase acts by a double displacement mechanism, and the nucleophilic serine hydroxyl group of the enzyme attacks penicillin bound at the active site that leads to the formation of an inactivated, penicillinoylated enzyme.DD transpeptidase is important for cross-linkage in cell wall synthesis of Gram-positive bacteria. Thus, the cell loses its wall (a cell without cell wall is called protoplast). On the other hand, gram-negative bacteria cells do not lose their cell wall completely and are called spheroplasts. In both cases, cells undergo lysis due to osmotic pressure. Ampicillin attacks both gram-negative and gram-positive organisms. Penicillin-resistant bacteria inactivate penicillin by the cleavage of the four-membered β-lactam ring of natural penicillins. Penicillin and related antibiotics are inactivated by β-lactamases, whereas chloramphenicol is inactivated by acylation on one or both of the hydroxyl groups.

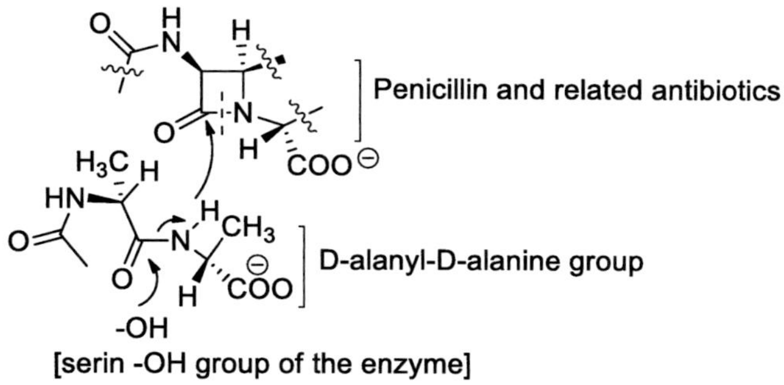

Being on the safe side, we must not use antibiotics randomly until or unless it is mandatory. Antibiotics lead to mutation of genes that, in turn, inactivate the antibiotic. In addition, over use of antibiotics causes resistance *e.g.*, minor infection treatment or wide spread use on the farm. With the rapid development of resistance, scientists are relentlessly developing the antibiotic either *via* a semi-synthetic pathway or identifying a new class of antibiotics. One such antibiotic is Vancomycin, which prevents crosslinking like penicillin but is unaffected by β-lactamases.

Why different types of penicillins are required is a commonly asked question. Their very similar structures means that their properties, including their antibacterial spectrum, as well as any bacterial resistance to them, will almost be identical. There are several factors that determine these issues.

- **Number of Possible Routes of Administration**: Acid stable penicillins, such as dicloxacillin, flucloxacillin, phenoxymethylpenicillin, and amoxicillin, are most suited for oral administration. Aqueous soluble penicillins, such as, piperacillin and ticarcillin, have been developed for injection alongside β-lactamase inhibitors to allow rapid treatment of life-threatening infections, such as, septicaemia and peritonitis.

- **Enhancing Bioavailability and Decreasing Side Effects**: Poor oral bioavailable prodrug esters, for example pivmecillinam, are employed to enhance the absorption of drugs due to their zwitterionic nature.

- **Having Agents with Different Antibacterial Spectra**: Variation in the C-6 amide R1 group can be used to obtain penicillins with a different antibacterial spectrum; for example, piperacillin has an extended spectrum of activity like Gram-positive and negative organisms, while ticarcillin is active only against Gram-negative organisms.

Commercial production of penicillin is very demanding with the increasing needs. One such protocol is the penicillin V synthesis from the phthalimide derivative of malate by Sheehan and Henerey-Logan in 1959. This is condensed with a suitable amino acid with the formation of a thiazolidine unit. Phthalimide is chopped with hydrazine to get a free amino acid. The free amino group is then acylated and hydrolyzed to di-acid. This di-acid is condensed internally to get penicillin V.

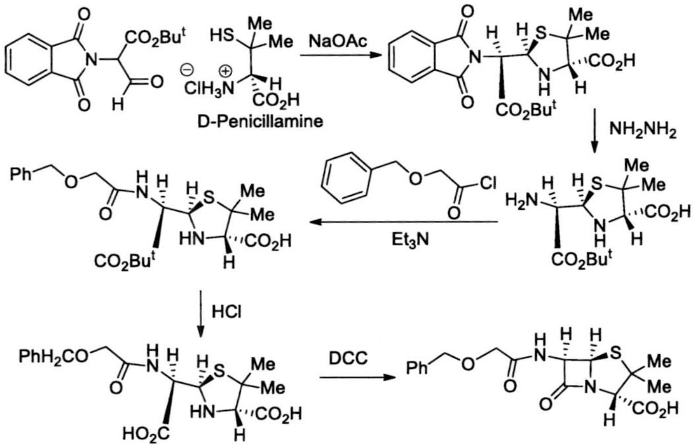

The fermentation of Penicillin G into 6-aminopenicillanic acid (6-APA) by enzyme penicillin acylase made it useful for the template development of semi-synthetic penicillins with better antimicrobial activity.

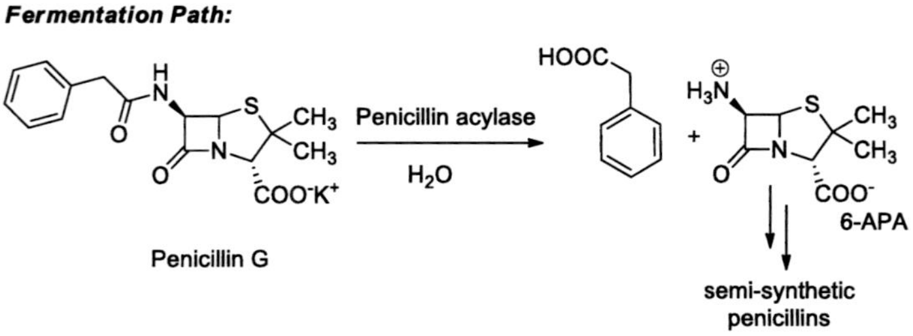

The biocatalyst, 6-APA, is also chemically developed from Penicillin G *via* several steps, but the economically preferred route is the enzyme-catalyzed reaction. The 6-APA is an important precursor to penicillin and cephalosporin antibiotics development against drug-resistant bacteria.

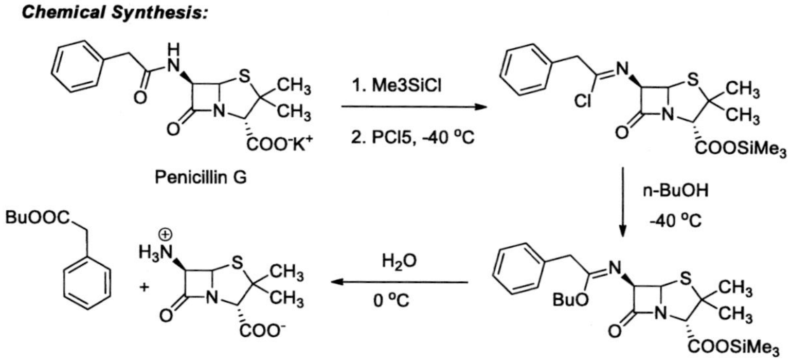

A number of modified penicillins, amino acids, vitamins, fructose syrup, and biopharmaceuticals are obtained by this method. Amoxicillin, used to treat different types of infections caused by bacteria, such as tonsillitis, bronchitis, pneumonia, and infections of the ear, nose, throat, skin, or urinary tract, is one of the easiest to synthesize from 6-APA and makes it a cheaper pathway.

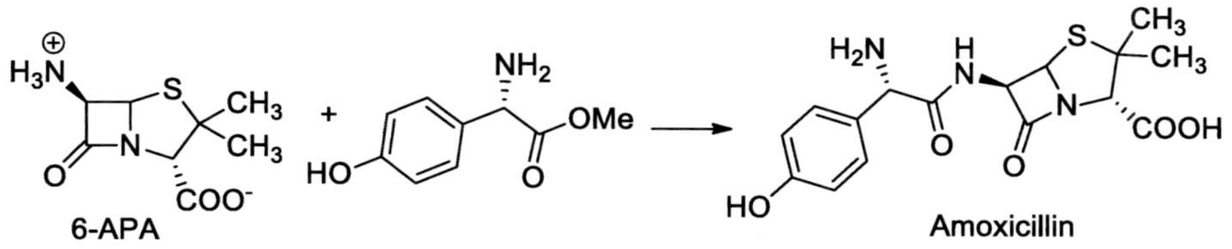

Fermentation

Important steps for the fermentation of penicillin:

1. **Fermentation medium**: Fermentation medium is prepared to obtain a sufficient amount of carbon source, nitrogen source, nutrients, aminoacids, salts, and precursors. This medium is useful for the growth of mycelium, accumulation, extraction, and purification of penicillin.

Carbon Source	Glucose, Lactose, and Sucrose
Nitrogen source	Ammonium sulphate, Ammonium acetate, Ammonium lactate
Amino acids	Corn steep liquor
Precursors for penicillin G	Phenylacetic acid

Precursors for penicillin X	Hydroxyphenylacetic acid
Precursors for penicillin V	Phenoxyacetic acid

2. **Fermentation organism**: In the early age, *Penicillium notatum* strain was used for the fermentation of penicillin, but due to its low efficiency, *Penicillium chrysogenumis* being used for a better yield. The latter has also been improved with genetic mutation technology for a high yielding product.

3. **Inoculum preparation**: The pure culture of *Penicillium chrysogenum* is prepared in sufficient amount for the production of penicillin. The pure culture is then added to special agar, which provides sporulation of spores. The sporulated spores are suspended in sodium lauryl sulphonate in a proportion of 1:10,000 approximately. Now, these spores are added in a nutrient medium of wheat bran plus nutrient. This flask is incubated for 5 to 7 days at 24 °C and is used as an inoculum in the fermentation tank.

4. **Fermentation process**: Fermentation is carried out either in trays or by submerged culture method. The 10 % of inoculum is added in the fermentor, maintaining the temperature at 25 °C to 26 °C, and sterile air supply is provided continuously. The fermentation generally took about 3 to 5 days. The fermentation process is monitored by collecting samples aseptically and is checked for yield, pH, and contamination. Checking of contamination is very important as contaminated organisms cause a great economic loss to the industry by producing some unwanted products. The fermentation process is also monitored for foam formation by an antifoaming agent.

Another parameter is pH, which initially remains constant since the inoculum utilizes carbon as a source of energy, but with time, the concentration of carbon reduces and the microorganism starts utilization of nitrogen as a source of energy. At this point, deamination causes a release of ammonia and ultimately pH of the fermentation media increases from 7.0 to 7.5. Momentarily, microorganisms start product synthesis by utilization of lactose and production of penicillin. After product formation, the concentration of lactose is decreased and pH rises to 8 or higher, which results in autolysis of mycelium. Thus, the fermentation is stopped and the recovery product is started. The usual yield obtained is 3 % to 5 %, with about 1500 units per milliliter of fermentation medium.

5. **Recovery and harvest of penicillin**: The mycelium and other solid suspended particles are removed by the filtration process. Phosphoric acid and sulphuric

acid are added to the filtrate such that the pH of the medium becomes 2-3 and then extracted with solvent butyl acetate. Penicillin, in an organic solvent, is extracted in water by using potassium hydroxide (pH ~6) in the form of salt.The aqueous penicillin is evaporated and crystallized in the form of the potassium salt of penicillin.

Commercial Production

Anaerobic fermentation is used for the commercial production of penicillin by a submerged aerated fermentation process. Commercial penicillin is produced by the stain *Penicillium chrysogenum*, developed using mutagenesis and recombinant technology. This production is carried out in a Fed-batch reactor with an approximate volume of 25000-60000 gallons. The main carbon source is glucose from molasses and the nitrogen source is corn steep liquor. The optimum temperature for the process is 25 °C and the pH is maintained between 6.4-6.8. A membrane filter is used to aerate the process such that the dissolved oxygen is 30%. The time of fermentation is nearly 120-200h. For the production of penicillin V and penicillin G, phenoxyacetic acid and phenylacetic acid are, respectively, being used.

Separation is done by membrane filtration, which separates the insoluble from the liquor. The mycelium is rewashed with distilled water to get trapped in penicillin. The liquor is maintained at pH 2-2.5 and extracted with butyl acetate. The organic layer is further extracted with buffer solution (pH 6.0) and penicillin rich buffer solution is again extracted with butyl acetate to get high potency penicillin. The penicillin is recrystallized using K-acetate to isolate as K-salt.

CEPHALOSPORIN

Cephalosporins are a large group of broad-spectrum β-lactam antibiotics [5, 6]. They are bactericidal and have the same mode of action as that of other β-lactam antibiotics. They are used to treat a wide variety of bacterial infections, such as respiratory tract infections, skin infections, and urinary tract infections. This is not a first choice antibiotic but used when others like penicillins do not work. Since the discovery of this antibiotic in the year 1945, its structure is being modified to make it broader and each modification gave a new generation of cephalosporins. There are five generations of cephalosporins and these start with cef, ceph, or kef.

1st generation	Cefadroxil, Cephalexin, Cefazolin, *etc.*	Active against gram-positive bacteria such as *staphylococci* and *streptococci*. They have little activity against gram-negative bacteria.
2nd generation	Cefotetan, Cefoxitin, Cefprozil, Cefuroxime *etc.*	Active against gram-negative bacteria, with less activity against gram-positive bacteria.
3rd generation	Ceftazidime, Cefotaxime, Cefpodoxime, Ceftriaxone, *etc.*	This followed the second-generation cephalosporins. No single third-generation cephalosporin treats all infectious diseases.
4th generation	Cefclidine, Cefepime, Cefpirome, *etc.*	Structurally similar to 3rd generation but with one extra ammonium group. Active against β-lactamase producing *Enterobacteriaceae,* which may inactivate third-generation cephalosporins.
5th generation	Ceftarolinem, Ceftobiprole, Ceftolozane, *etc.*	Active against methicillin-resistant *Staphylococcus aureus* and gram-positive bacteria.

Cephalosporin C is closely related to penicillin's structure. It contains a D-α-amino adipoyl side chain and is replaced to form various semi-synthetic cephalosporins. An enzyme deacetoxycephalosporin C synthase convert spenicillins into cephalosporins. Similar to penicillin, δ-(L-α-aminoadipoyl)-L-cysteinyl-D-valine synthetase forms the precursor to cephalosporins [43f].

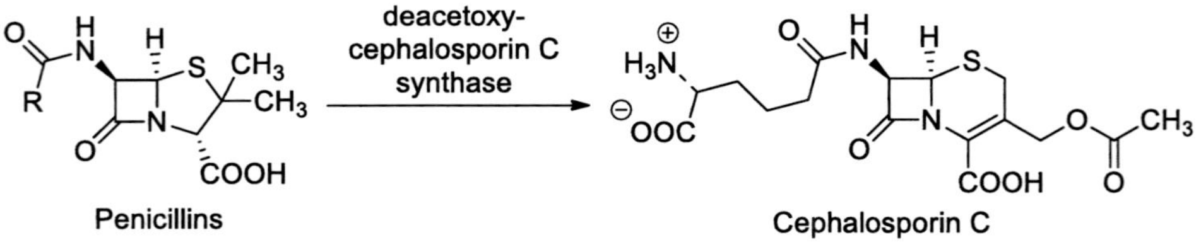

Similar to 6-APA, 7-aminocephalosporanic acid (7-ACA) is produced from cephalosporin *via* chemical degradation [43f]. Over decades, 7-ACA, as a key intermediate, has been developed economically and ecologically for the large scale manufacture of β-lactam-type antibiotic drugs. Isogai *et al.* showed that D-amino acid oxidase (DAO) and glutarylacylase (GLA) are used biosynthetically for preparing 7-ACA from the alkaline protease gene of *Acremonium chrysogenum.* They claimed that *cephalosporin acylase* could directly convert the cephalosporin

C into 7-ACA, but the yield is low.There are a number of chemical reactions that can be used for this purpose.

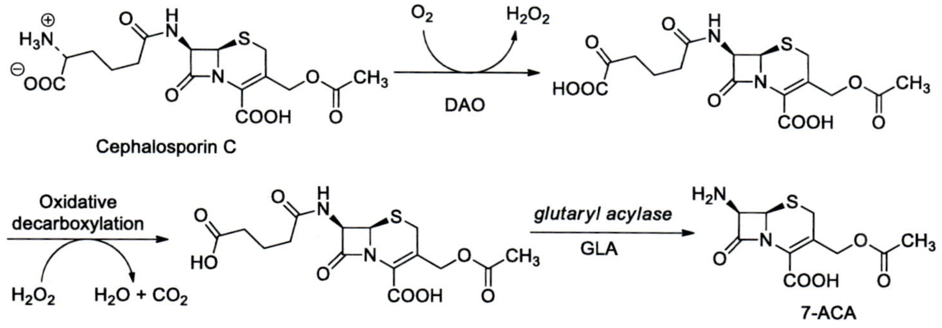

From this 7-ACA, many cephalosporins are synthesized, keeping its main structural skeleton intact.

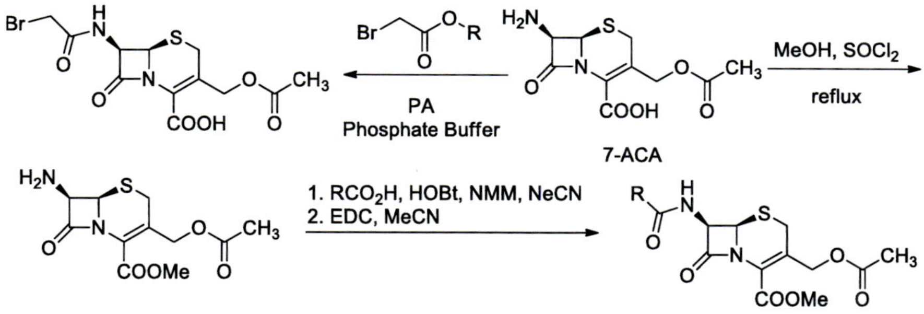

Therefore, industrially, 6-APA and 7-ACA were used to produce their derivatives, such as 6-substituted penicillin and 3 and 7-substituted cephalosporin based antibiotics, respectively [43g].

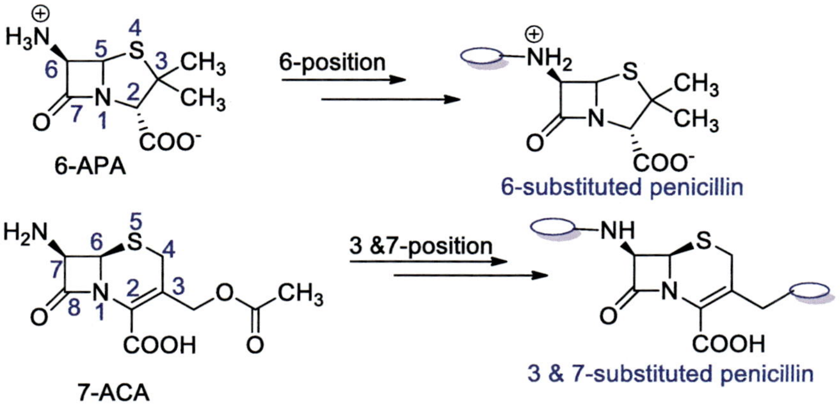

Chloromycetin

Chloramphenicol is a man-made antibiotic and marketed under many brand names. Chloromycetin is used in ophthalmic treatment as an ointment. It works by killing bacteria or preventing their growth. Each gram of Chloromycetin Ophthalmic Ointment, 1% contains 10 mg of chloramphenicol in a special base of liquid petrolatum and polyethylene.

Streptomycin

Streptomycin, a trisaccharide, was isolated from soil *actinomycetes* (streptomyces) by Waksman. Streptomycin, the neomycins, paromomycin, gentamycin, and kanamycin have one structural unit in common. This falls into aminoglycoside antibiotics and is effective against tuberculosis caused by *Mycobacterium tuberculi*. Streptomycin causes ribosomes to misread the genetic code and consequently inhibits protein synthesis. The strong water solubility is due to three sugar units in its structure and derived from D-Glucose. Streptomycin is inactivated by enzymes catalyzing phosphorylation or adenylation of hydroxyl groups on the sugar rings. Streptomycin is active against Gram (-) negative bacteria and particularly useful in the treatment of infections caused by Gram (+) ve bacteria, especially resistant to penicillin [6, 37]. Use of higher dose may cause neurotoxicity, such as hearing impairment and loss of balance maintenance in man. However, dihydro-streptomycin shows decreased activity. For this reason, dihydrostreptomycin is produced.

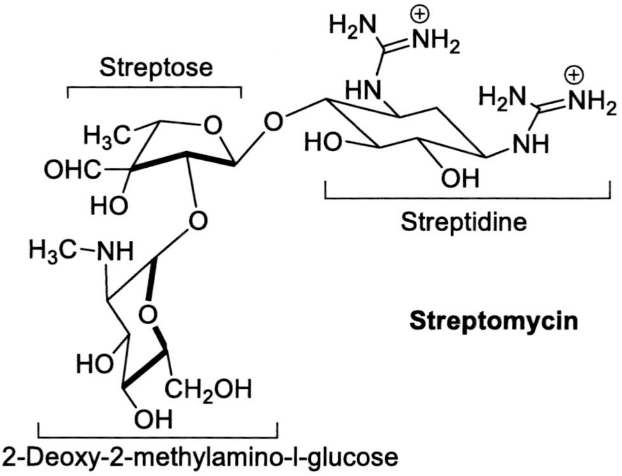

Streptomycin

Biosynthesis

Metabolism of sugar produces the ketone group *via* the oxidation of the hydroxyl group. Biosynthesis of streptose and streptidine part is known, but 2-deoxy-2-methylamino-L-glucose is not clear. It is expected that about 28 enzymes take part in the conversion of glucose into streptomycin (Fig. **1**) [43a-c].

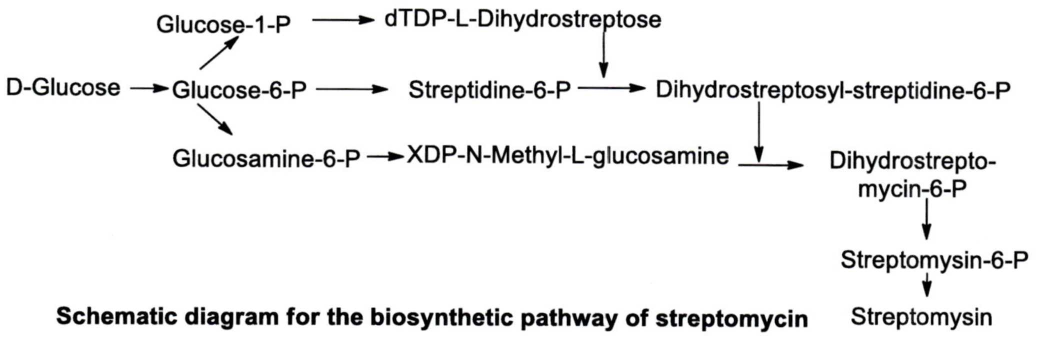

Fig. (1). Schematic diagram for the biosynthetic pathway of streptomycin.

Streptose synthesis: The intermediate of the L-rhamnose synthesis from D-glucose *i.e.*, nucleoside diphosphate (dTDP: deoxythymidine diphosphate) sugar, acts as a starting material for streptose synthesis. The carbon–carbon chain undergoes an aldol cleavage followed by recyclization *via* aldol condensation to form a five-membered ring with a branch at C-3 position *i.e.*, Streptosyl-TDP [3].

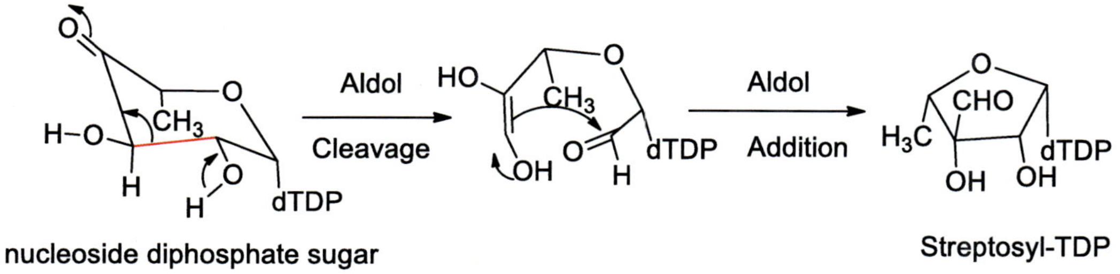

Streptidine synthesis: Streptidine is derived from *myo*-inositol. *myo*-inositol is produced from glucose 6-P. It's appropriate hydroxyl group is oxidized to the carbonyl group and then aminated *via* trans-amination from a specific amino donor so as to install guanidino groups. Glutamine is the amino donor for the trans-amination, the oxo-acid product being α-oxoglutaramic acid. Then amine is converted to amidine group in the presence of arginine. Phosphatase hydrolyzed the phosphate group. The second oxidation at the 3 position followed by transamination by alanine gives an amine group. Theamine group is then converted into a guanidine group from arginine.

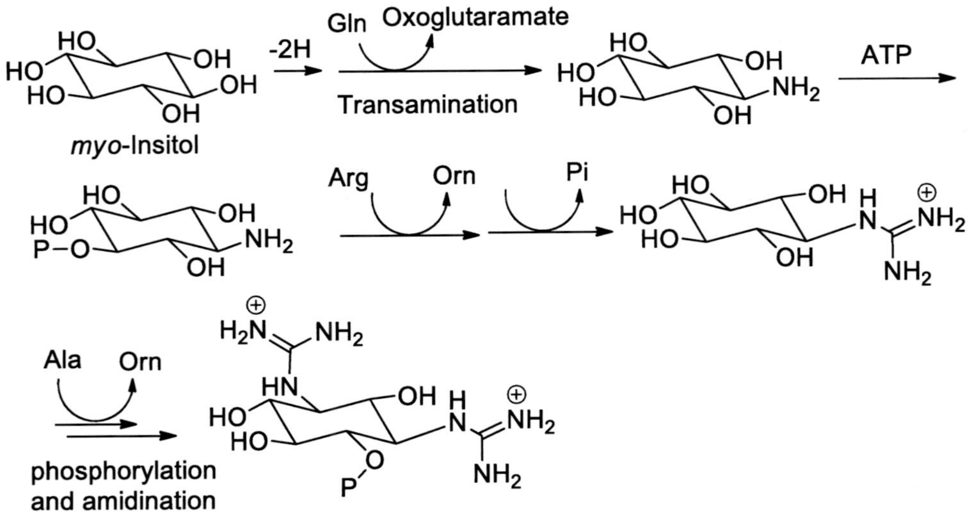

Fermentation

Industrially, streptomycin is produced by submerged culture method,

(a) The Inoculum Production: The spores of S. griseus from the stock cultures are transferred to a sporulation medium to provide enough sporulated growth to initiate liquid culture build-up of mycelial inoculum in inoculum tanks. When mycelial growth is sufficient, it is fed to the production fermenter [43d].

(b) Preparation of the Medium: A medium containing glucose as the main carbon source as well as peptones, soya extract, meat extract, the residue from alcohol distillation, ammonium salts, nitrates, and glycine as a nitrogen source, is prepared. Apart from glucose, fructose, maltose, lactose, galactose, mannitol, xylose, and starch can also be used as carbon sources. Magnesium, calcium, potassium, boron, and molybdenum may be used as mineral sources along with sulphates, phosphates, and chlorides. To obtain a better yield, phenylacetic acid and L-naphthalene acetic acid are also added as growth stimulating compounds. The presence of proline into the medium helps in high streptomycin production.

(c) Fermentation: The sterilized liquid medium is then fed to the production fermenter. The fermentor contains 4-5% volume with inoculum. The temperature of the fermentation is maintained between 25 to 30 °C and the pH ranges between 7.0 and 8.0. The process is highly aerobic and lasts for approximately 5 to 7 days. Fermentation is carried out in 3 phases:

- **The First Phase:** This phase is associated with rapid growth and the formation of abundant mycelium takes place within 24 hours to 48 hours. The pH becomes 8.0 due to the release of ammonia into the medium

- **The Second Phase:** In this step, streptomycin production takes place without an increase in the mycelial growth and lasts for 2 days. The pH of the medium decreases to 7.6-8.0 as ammonia produced in the 1st phase is consumed. Sufficient glucose and oxygen are necessary for this phase.

- **Third Phase:** In this phase, pH increases again as cells undergo lysis and ammonia is released. Finally, streptomycin production ceases. In this process, streptomycin is obtained at 1200 micrograms per milliliter.

(d) Harvest and Recovery: After the completion of fermentation, the mycelium is separated from the broth by filtration. The most acceptable method for streptomycin isolation involves the following commonly used steps: The fermentation broth is acidified, filtered, and neutralized. It is then passed through a column containing a cation exchange resin to adsorb the streptomycin from the broth. The column is then washed with water and the antibiotic is eluted with hydrochloric acid or cyclohexanol or phosphoric acid. It is then concentrated at about 60 °C under vacuum. The streptomycin is then dissolved in methanol and filtered and acetone is added to the filtrate to precipitate the antibiotic. The precipitate is again washed with acetone and vacuum dried. It is purified further by dissolving in methanol. The streptomycin in pure form is extracted as a calcium chloride complex.

(e) By-product Vitamin B_{12}: Vitamin B_{12} is produced as a by product that will not adversely affect the yield of streptomycin.

From Streptonzyces Griseus

Streptonzyces griseus is extensively distributed in soils, peats, and composts. Few strains of this organism are capable of producing streptomycin and mostly produce no antibiotic at all. Culture, belonging to *Streptonzyces griseus*, is grown in nutrient and corn steep broths, a very few of these are found to be capable of producing streptomycin [43d]. Culture is grown both in stationary and in submerged cultures. The submerged culture undergoes rapid, even if incomplete, lysis in 3 to 5 days.

Media containing meat extract or corn steep, but free from glucose, gave the best activity. The agar streak method is used. The results point to a very narrow antibiotic spectrum, which is not limited either to the gram- positive or to the gram-negative bacteria. The culture filtrate is treated with 5 g activated charcoal (per liter) to remove the entire antibiotic. On the treatment of the charcoal with 9% ethanol, almost half of the total activity was recovered. The eluated alcohol is concentrated to syrup, and dehydrated methanol was added till a precipitate began to form. The final preparation is precipitated with acetone, washed with ether, and desiccated. From the one literculture,400-600mg antibioticis obtained.

From Streptomyces Bikiniensis

Streptomyces bikiniensis is cultured in the same broth that is commonly used for the production of streptomycin [43e]. This broth contains 3 g meat exract, 5 g peptone, 10 g glucose, and 5 g NaCl per liter water. The cultures are incubated at 28 °C in both static and shaken conditions. Some of the cultures are removed after definite incubation periods and filtered through paper.The filtrates were tested by the agar streak method (Waksman and Reilly, 1945). The static cultures are some what more satisfactory than the shaken cultures for the growth of *S. bikiniensis* and for the production of the antibiotic. The shaken cultures gave greater activity in a shorter time. This activity is not as high as in the static cultures and soon tend to disappear completely. The antibacterial spectrum of the culture filtrates appeared in both cases, however, to be very similar to that of streptomycin.

The antibiotic produced by *S. bikinienaisis* isolated from the culture medium by the method commonly employed for the isolation of streptomycin. The active material is readily removed from the culture filtrate by adsorption on it. The adsorbate is washed with neutral alcohol and treated with acidified ethyl alcohol. The alcoholic extract is filtered, neutralized, and the alcohol is driven off by distillation at low temperatures. The residue is dried in vacuo. The active material is precipitated directly from the alcoholic solution by the addition of several volumes of acetone. It is also isolated by various procedures commonly used in the isolation of streptomycin, such as the methyl-alcohol formic acid method. Preparations are, thus, obtained that had an activity of 30 to 50 units per milligram, comparable to the streptomycin yields obtained by similar procedures in the early studies with *Streptomyces griseus*.

CHAPTER 9

Production of Amino Acids and Vitamins

Abstract: In this chapter, commercial fermentation process of amino acids like Lysine, Glutamic acid and vitamins like Vitamin B2, Vitamin B12, and Vitamin C have discussed. Their importance, metabolic precursor for commercial production described in a simple way.

Keywords: Drug discovery, Pharmaceuticals, Pharmaceutical chemistry, Pharmacology, Pharmacokinetics.

PRODUCTION OF AMINO ACIDS

Amino acids and vitamins including minerals are useful nutrients for the normal body growth of animals. Human's body cannot synthesize all vitamins and amino acids [39, 40]. The amino acid tryptophan is used for niacin synthesis. Amino acids are obtained from intermediates in glycolysis, the citric acid cycle, or the pentose phosphate pathway. Nitrogen comes from glutamate and glutamine. Most of the bacteria and plants can easily synthesize 20 amino acids. Ten of the amino acids are obtained easily, while the aromatic amino acids are more complex. Plants synthesize almost all the amino acids, but animals can synthesize half of them. Animals can do that in a very simple way and these are called non-essential amino acids. But the amino acids that cannot be synthesized and require for normal growth are known as essential amino acids – Metheonine, Threonine, Lysine, Isoleucine, Leucine, Valine, Tryptophan, Phenylalanine, Histidine. These come from the diet and are a source of plant. So, with the growing need, it is important to get practice for their commercial synthesis [38, 43d].

Based on the metabolic precursor of each amino acid, they were grouped into six-metabolic precursor (Table **1**) [37]. This clearly indicates that

1. **α-Ketoglutarate precursor group**: α-ketoglutarate produces Glutamate, Glutamine, Arginine, Proline;

2. **3-Phosphoglycerate precursor group**: 3-phosphoglycerate produces Serine, Glycine, Cysteine;

3. **Oxaloacetate precursor group**: Oxaloacetate produces Aspartate, Asparagine, Methonine, Threonine, Lysine, Isoleucine;

Samir Kumar Mandal and Rebeca Ghanta (Eds.)

4. **Pyruvate precursor group**: Pyruvate produces Alanine, Leucine, Valine;

5. **Phosphoenolpyruvate precursor group**: Phosphoenolpyruvate and erythose-4-phosphate produces Tryptophan, Phenylalanine, Tyrosine;

6. **Ribose-5-phosphate precursor group**: Ribose-5-phosphate produces Histidine.

Table 1. Metabolic precursor of amino acids.

Precursor	Amino Acid	Abbreviation	Structure
α-ketoglutarate	1. Glutamate	Glu	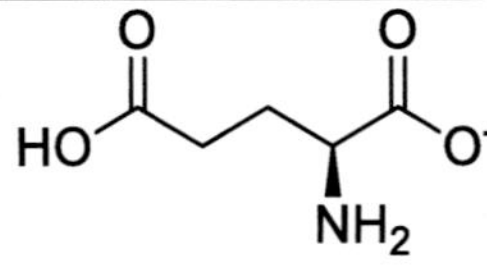
	2. Glutamine	Gln	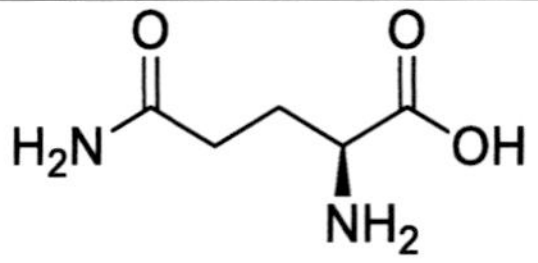
	3. Arginine	Arg	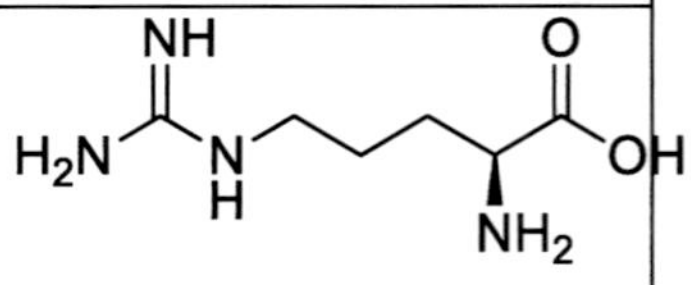
	4. Proline	Pro	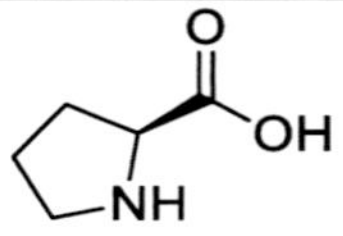
3-phosphoglycerate	5. Serine	Ser	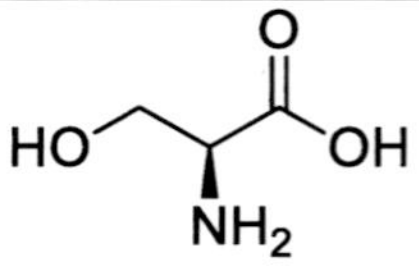
	6. Glycine	Gly	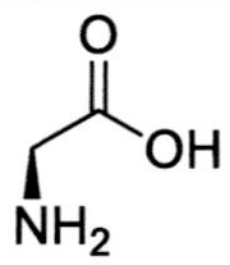

Precursor	**Amino Acid**	**Abbreviation**	**Structure**
	7. Cysteine	Csy	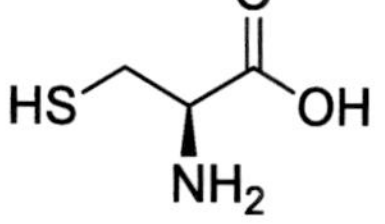
Oxaloacetate	8. Aspartate	Asp	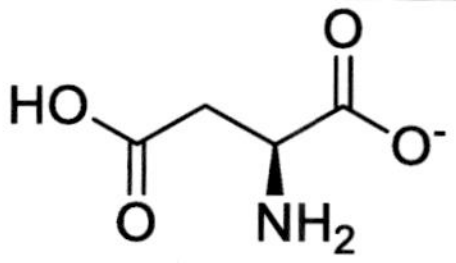
	9. Asparagine	Asn	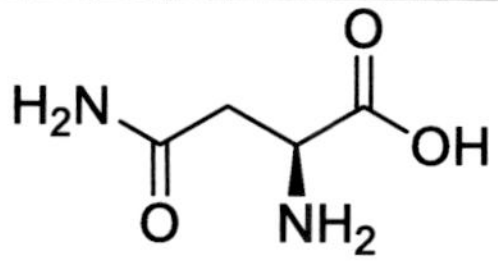
	10. Methonine	Met	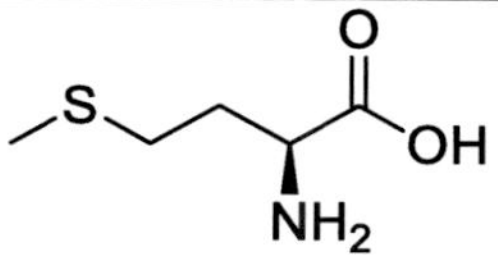
	11. Threonine	Thr	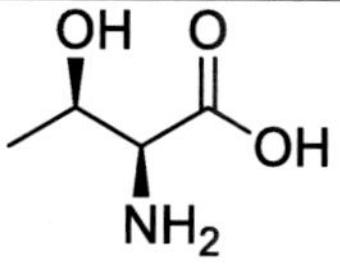
	12. Lysine	Lys	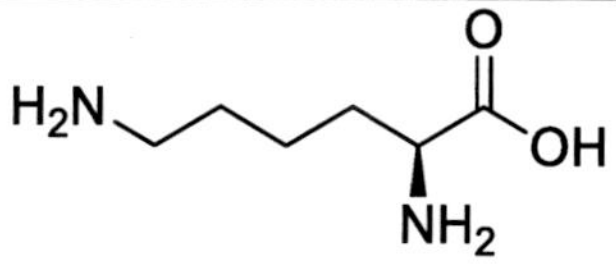
	13. Isoleucine	Ile	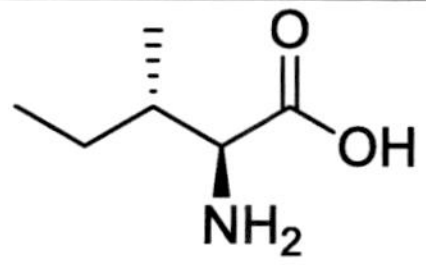
Pyruvate	14. Alanine	Ala	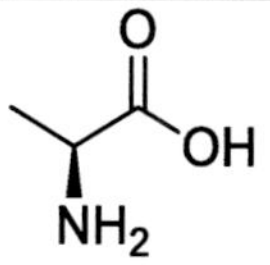

Precursor	Amino Acid	Abbreviation	Structure
	15. Leucine	Leu	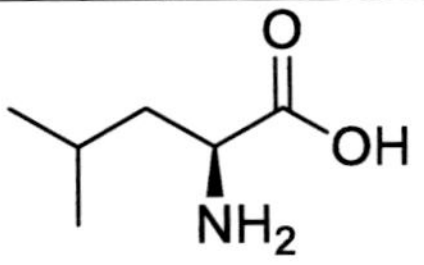
	16. Valine	Val	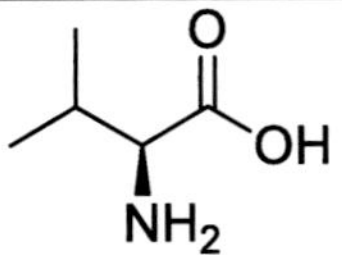
Phosphoenolpyruvate and erythose-4-phosphate	17. Tryptophan	Trp	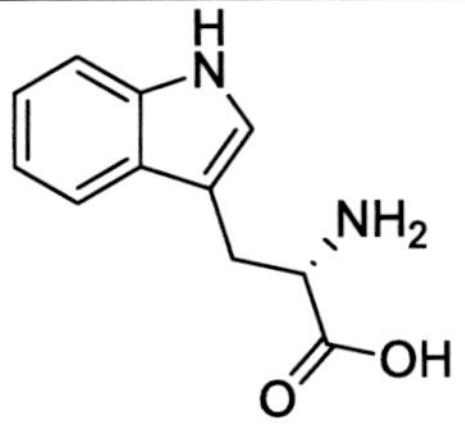
	8. Phenyl-alanine	Phe	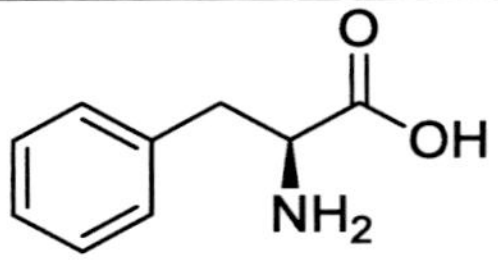
	19. Tyrosine	Tyr	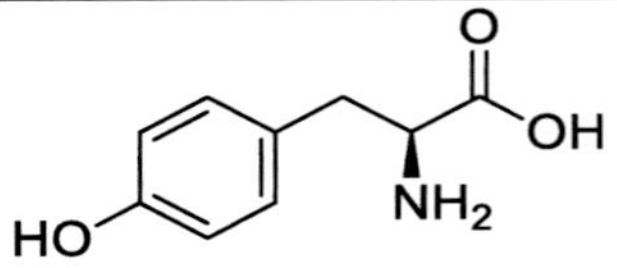
Ribose-5-phosphate	20. Histidine	His	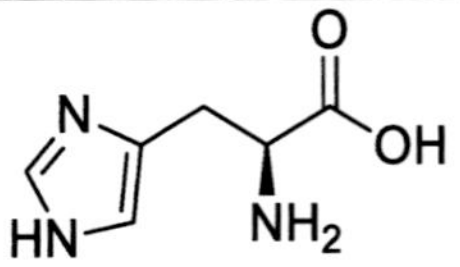

LYSINE

Lysine is an essential (human body cannot synthesize) α-amino acid used for preventing and treating cold sores. Thus, it prevents the growth of the herpes virus. Other than this, it helps to protect from cold sores, shingles, and human papillomavirus (HPV). This is useful for protein synthesis in the living system and, in many cases, used as nutritional supplements to protect muscle deterioration [44].

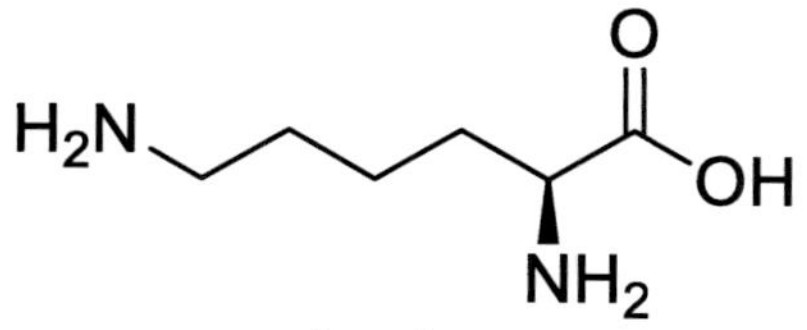

Lysine

Lysine is synthesized from α-amino adipic acid by yeast and from diaminopimalic acid by *E. Coli*.

Lysine	
Precursor	α-amino adipic acid (Oxaloacetate precursor group)
Microorganism	*E. Coli*
pH	7
Temperature	30 °C
Time	~96h

In a fermentative process, starches, molasses, glucose are used as carbon source and the ratio of carbon and nitrogen are maintained by using corn steep liquor, soyabean cake acid hydrolysate, yeast extract, peptone, *etc.* Salts required as nutrients are $(NH_4)_2SO_4$, K_2HPO_4, KH_2PO_4, $MgSO_4$, $ZnSO_4$, $MnSO_4$ and $FeSO_4$. The optimum pH and temperature for this process are 7 and 30 °C, respectively. The time required for the fermentation process is around 96h.

The biosynthetic pathways for lysine are complex and interconnected. The synthetic path is even different for bacteria, fungi, and plants. The bacterial pathway is common.

In the synthetic pathway of bacteria, oxaloacetate produces aspartate [37]. Then, aspartate gives rise to methionine, threonine, and lysine *via* aspartate-β-semi-aldehyde as a common intermediate in all three different pathways. Aspartate-β-semialdehyde in the way of lysine synthesis produces dihydropicolinate, piperidine-2,6-dicarboxylate and differently substituted pimelate as intermediates.

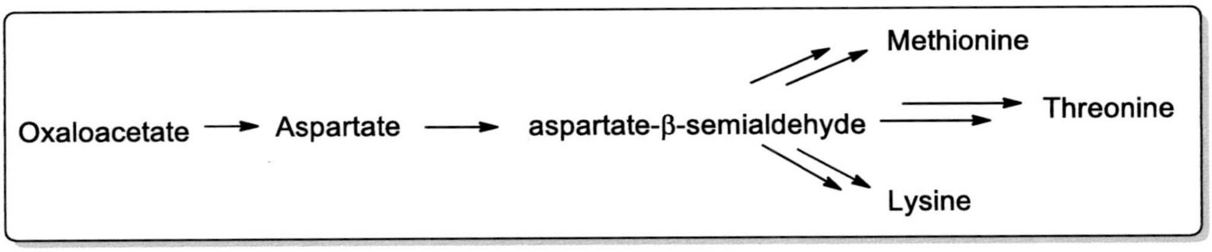

GLUTAMIC ACID

Glutamic acid is a non-essential α-amino acid and is used by living beings in the biosynthesis of proteins [37]. In human blood, it is the most abundant free amino acid. Commercially, its salt is very much useful in food industries for enhancing flavor. This is useful for peptic ulcer and muscle recovery. As a pharmaceutics, it is used importantly as a neurotransmitter. It is a useful precursor of GABA [3, 45].

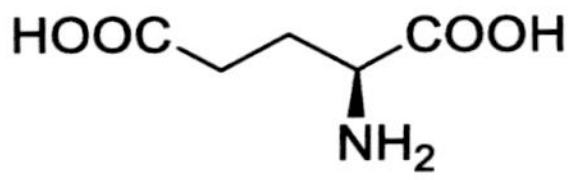

Glutamic acid

Glutamic acid can combine with N-methyl-D-aspartate (NMDA) receptor to increase cation conduction and depolarize the cell membrane and deblocking the NMDA receptor [3, 5].

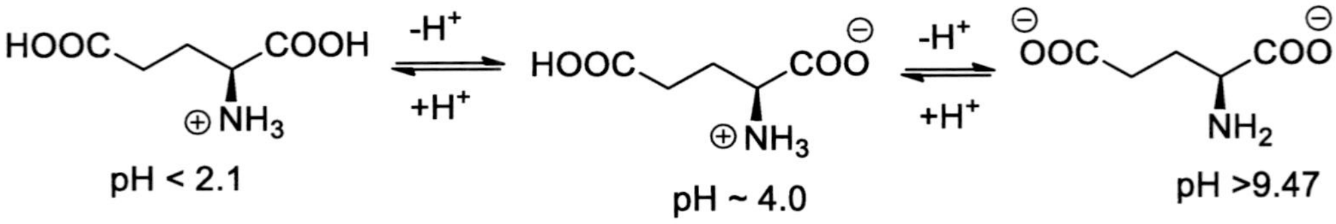

The most popular microorganisms involved in the production of glutamic acid are *Coryneform species e.g. C. Glutamium, Corynibacterium* and *Brevibacterium species e.g. Brevibacteriumr oseum, Brevibacterium lactofermentum, Brevi bacterium ammoniagenes, Brevibacterium sacchharoliticum, etc.* Other micro-organisms are *Eshcherichia coli, Basillus circulans, Basillus cereus*. Industrially glutamic acid is produced by a batch submerged fermentation process using genetically modified strains of *Coryneform species* and *Brevibacterium species* [37 38].

Glutamic Acid	
Precursor	α-Ketoglutarate
Microorganism	*Coryneform species*
pH	7
Temperature	30 °C
Time	~48h

In the fermentative process, the medium is prepared from glucose solution with corn steep liquor in a flask. To this solution, NH_4Cl, K_2HPO_4, KH_2PO_4, $MgSO_4$ and $CaCO_3$ were added along with deionised water. The pH of the medium is maintained at 7. For nitrogen, source urea is added. This medium is kept in incubator at 30 °C and inoculated. In the fermentor, molasses is added along with the nutrient. For fermentation, 48h aeration is continued along with agitation.

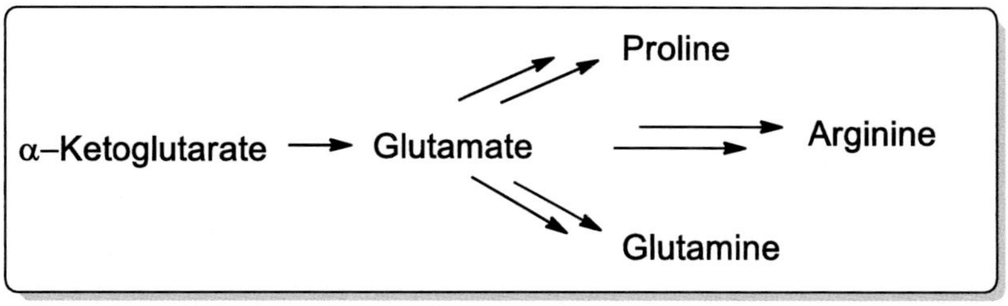

Both lysine and glutamic acid are produced from Krebs cycle, but intermediates are different. Lysine is produced from oxaloacetate and glutamic acid from α-ketoglutarate.

In bacteria, the enzyme glutamate synthase produces glutamate from α-ketoglutarate *via* reductive amination, where glutamine acts as a nitrogen donor. In animals, glutamate synthase is not known to occur (Fig. **1**) [37].

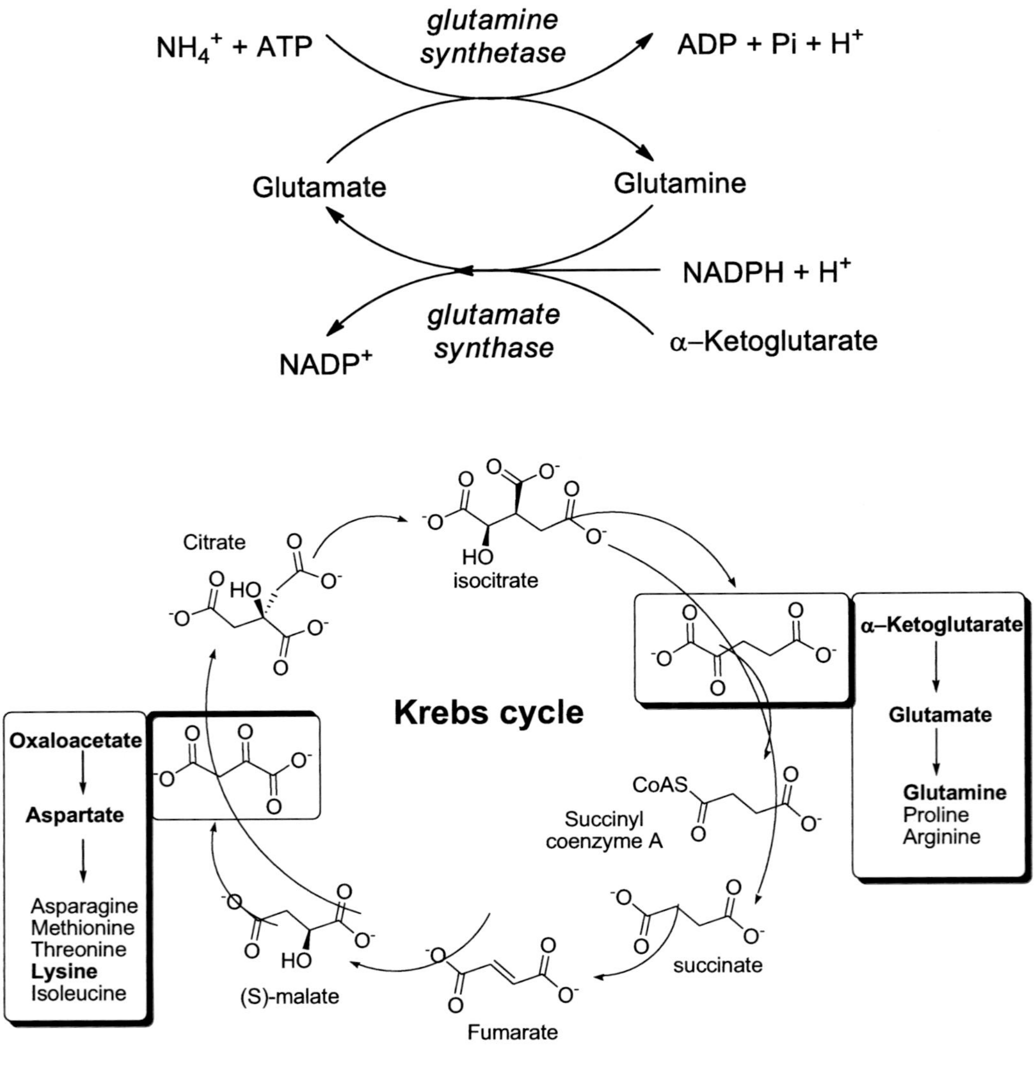

Fig. (1). Production of α- ketoglutarate.

The amino groups in most of the amino acids are the results of transamination reactions (Fig. **2**) and come from glutamate. While *glutamine synthetase* helps assimilation of ammonia with the formation of glutamine and there by decrease of toxic free ammonia level in blood. Then, the amide group of glutamine is used as the source of amino groups for many biosynthetic processes.

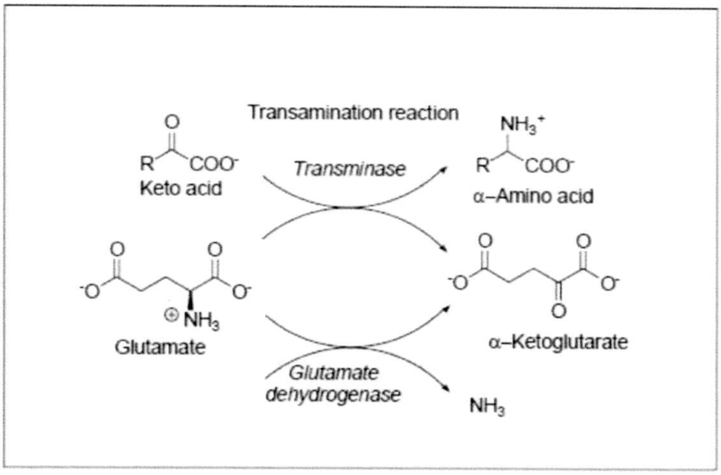

Fig. (2). Transamination reaction.

PRODUCTION OF VITAMIN

Vitamins are useful organic compounds for specific functions, *e.g.* metabolism of a living system [36]. They are not involved in the energy production rather assist the energy production reaction in the living cell. Humans can synthesize some of the vitamins, *e.g.* vitamin D is produced when the skin is exposed to sunlight. On the other hand,many bacteria living in the human gut cell can synthesize vitamin K and biotin (vitamin H). Niacin (vitamin B3) is synthesized from amino acid. Others are taken from different sources with food materials [5, 7, 35d].

Based on solubility, they are classified as fat soluble vitamins and water soluble vitamins. Fat soluble vitamins are Vitamin A, E, D, K and water soluble vitamins are Vitamin B, C, H, and P. Many of these are produced by a chemical breakdown of substances by yeasts/ bacteria/ other microorganisms known as fermentation. The common forms of vitamin B include vitamin B1 (thiamine), B2 (riboflavin), B3 (niacin), B6 (pyridoxine) and B12 (cyanocobalamin). Other than vitamin C, Vitamin E also acts as an antioxidant, thereby, protecting against free radical damage in lipid systems. Vitamin K plays a key role in blood clotting.

Vitamins derived from foods in precursor forms must be activated in the body before their function. For example, beta(β)-carotene, found in plants, is converted to vitamin A in the body.

Synthetic biology for the production of vitamin involves the following steps [38-39]:

Host Selection

Alpha-lipoic acid or ALA is a naturally occurring compound. It is made in the body. The host having the ability to supply precursors (ALA) and cofactors (*e.g.* S-adenosylmethionine) for the production of the desired chemical is important for this step. *Escherichia coli* is used to produce ALA in many studies, which is important for sufficient ALA supply for the vitamin B_{12} biosynthesis suggesting E. *coli* as a suitable host for vitamin B_{12} production. Due to the lack of genes involved in the cobalamin synthesis pathway, other bacteria are not suitable for this synthesis. Thus, *Escherichia coli* is a well-characterized prokaryote used as a microbial cell factory production of vitamin B12.

Gene Mining

In this step, enzyme activity is verified subsequently both in *in-vitro* and *in-vivo*. Spectroscopic analysis, mass spectrometry, or microbiological assays are used for assessment purposes.

Construction of Metabolic Pathway

Gene assembly methods such as Sequence- and Ligation-Independent Cloning (SLIC), Circular Polymerase Extension Cloning (CPEC), Gibson, golden gate, DNA assembler and Locus Control Region (LCR), or integrated into the genome methods are used for assembling the heterogeneous genes and other functional elements on plasmids.

Pathway Tuning

It is challenging to increase the flux of the intermediate to obtain the desired product. It is necessary to optimize gene expression in existing metabolic pathways to make it a highly evolved pathway.

Fermentation

The qualities of the engineered strains are verified *via* fermentation. Various substrates like ALA, cobalt ions, betaine and DMB and varying conditions like dissolved oxygen concentration, pH, and temperature can be optimized to improve yield and productivity.

VITAMIN B2 (RIBOFLAVIN)

Vitamin B2, also known as Riboflavin, is used for human nutrition and therapy. Its deficiency causes hair loss, skin inflammation and growth failure. In few cases, it is used to treat migraine and malaria [46]. Vitamin B2 is also important for red blood cell formation and respiration, antibody production, and reproduction. It is a precursor of the coenzymes flavin mononucleotide (FMN) and flavin adenine dinucleotide (FAD). These are important in normal tissue respiration, pyridoxine activation, tryptophan to niacin conversion, fat, carbohydrate, and protein metabolism, and glutathione reductase mediated detoxification. It is available in milk, eggs, malted barley, liver, kidney, heart, and leafy vegetables. Yeast is the richest source of vitamin B2. The free form of vitamin B2 is available in the retina of the eye, in whey, and in the urine.

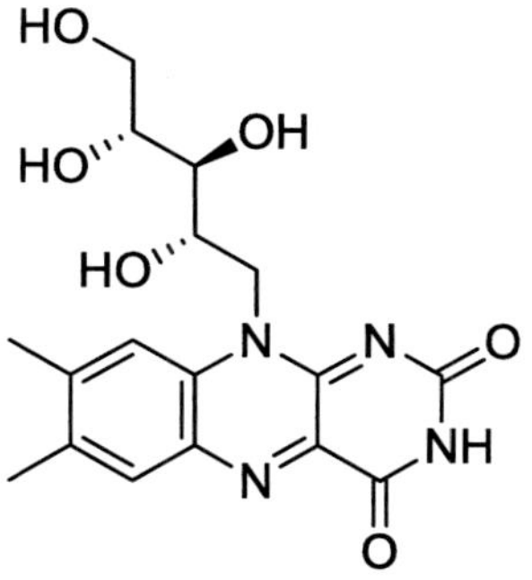

Riboflavin

7,8-dimethyl-10-[(2S,3S,4R)-2,3,4,5-tetrahydroxypentyl]benzo[g]pteridine-2,4-dione

This can be produced by fermentation and chemical processes. Bacteria (*Clostridium sp.*) and yeast (*Candida sp.*) are good to produce vitamin B2. Fungi namely, *Eremothecium ashbyii* and *Ashbya gossypi* are known to be the best producer of vitamin B2. Even later is much better as it produces 40000 times more than its growth. An improved stain is developed for its product through metabolic engineering *via* DNA recombinant technology in *Corynebacterium ammoniagenes*.

For the fermentation of vitamin B2, aerobic submerged process is used and medium is prepared from corn steep liquor/palm oil/molasses/soya oil as carbon source. Pure slant culture of *Ashbya gossypi* is inoculated and grown in inoculums medium. Then, it is incubated on a shaker to oxygenate the system. The cultures are used to inoculate large amount of inoculum medium kept in numbers of tanks [38, 39]. Medium pH is maintained around 6 to 7.5 and temperature around 26-28 °C. Aeration and agitation are kept at optimum level to avoid foaming. Fermentation time required in this process is around 100 hours. Vitamin B2 is recovered from the broth after the inactivation of the microorganism by heat. Centrifugation of the inactivated broth leads to the separation of cells and the riboflavin as their size and sedimentation behavior is different. Riboflavin obtained this way is dried under vacuum. This way 3-5 g vitamin B2 is produced per litre of the fermentation broth.

VITAMIN B12 (COBALAMIN)

Vitamin B12, known as cyanocobalamin, is a water soluble vitamin that plays an important role in the normal functioning of the nervous system and its daily required amount is 0.001 mg/day. Vitamin B12 improves iron functions in the metabolic cycle and assists folic acid in choline synthesis. Deficiency of vitamin B12 causes pernicious anemia, megaloblastic anemia, and neurologic lesions. Cyanocobalamin is generated by intestinal microbes. This vitamin is necessary for hematopoiesis, DNA and RNA production, and carbohydrate, fat, and protein metabolism.

This belongs to the cobalamin family of compounds, in which cobalt atom at the centre is surrounded with corrinoid ring composed of four pyrrol moieties and capped with upper 5,6-dimethyl benzimidazole and lower ligand (R= methyl or hydroxy or a cyano group). Cyanocobalamin is the stable form of Cobalamin, which is not found in nature [47].

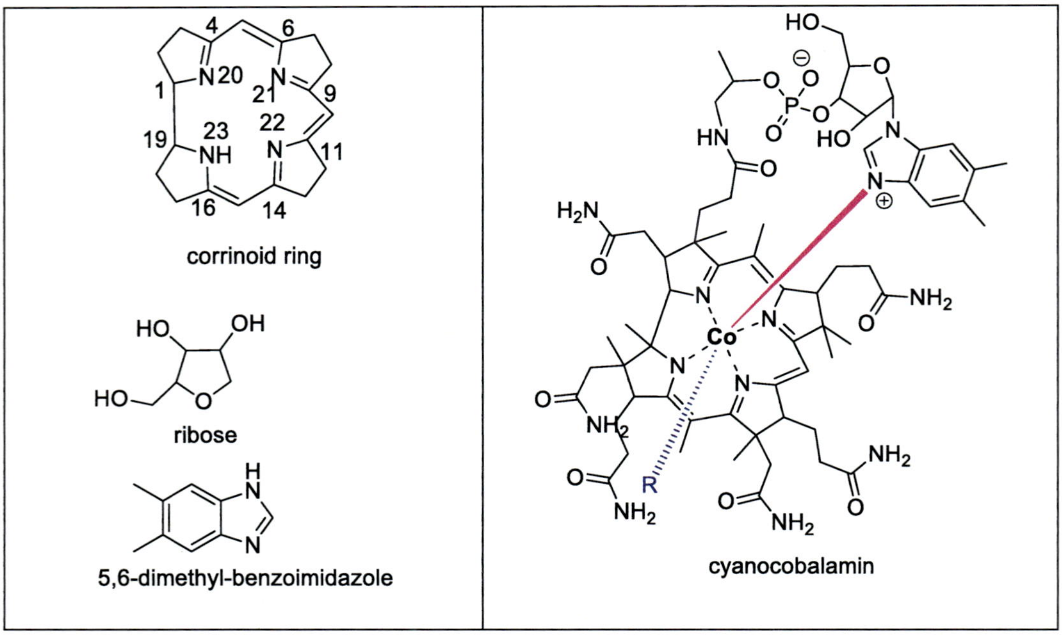

Synthetic biology is an efficient tool for the production of vitamin B12, selecting a suitable host. Thus, rational strain engineering is important to improve product yield. For fermentation of vitamin B12 *Streptomyces griseus, Pseudomonas denitrificans, Streptomyces olivaceus and Propionibacterium shermanii* are used as microorganism. *Pseudomonas denitrificans, Bacillus megaterium,* and *Propionibacterium freudenreichii* are used for commercial production [36, 39].

For the fermentation of vitamin B12, the medium is prepared from corn steep liquor and glucose as a carbon source. Pure slant culture of *Streptomyces Olivaceus NRRL B-1125* is inoculated and grown in inoculums medium. Then, *S. olivaceus* inoculation from the slant culture is done in the flask usually 100-250 ml of inoculums medium and then incubated on a shaker to oxygenate the system. The cultures are used to inoculate large amount of inoculum medium kept in a number of tanks. Ammonium phosphate or ammonium hydroxide is used for nitrogen source. Cobalt salt, hexaaquacobalt (II) chloride in 1-10 ppm, is added to maximise the yield of cobalamin and then sterilized in an autoclave with 15 lbs pressure at 121 °C. Now, fermentation is done by batch mode process. Initially, pH falls below 2 due to the consumption of glucose and then rises to 2-4 due to lysis of mycelium [5]. Medium pH 5 is maintained using sulfuric acid. Nutrients and inoculums are then added to the sterile fermenter and then left. Aeration and agitation were kept at an optimum level to avoid foaming. Now corn oil or soyabean/corn oil is used as anti-foaming agent. When a good amount of product is present in the fermenter, the content is then taken out and the product is extracted. The culture broth contains 10-15 mg Vitamin B12 per litre. To get a concentrated amount of mass of cells, the culture broth is then centrifuged. The impurities are separated from the culture medium using vacuum filtration. The cell mass is treated with a dilute acid maintaining the temperature of around 10-30 °C. Now cyanide solution is added to separate 5,6-dimethyl benzimidazolecobalamide and pseudovitamin B12, as a result of which Vitamin B12 (cyanocobalamine) is then released in solution. Vitamin B12, which is in the liquid form is then separated by adsorption column chromatography process. Phenolic solvent is used to remove the adsorbed cyanocobalamine in the column and the solvent is removed by evaporation to get crystaline cyanocobalamine. This way 1-2 mg vitamin B12 is produced per litre of the fermentation broth.

Biosynthesis

Synthesis of Vitamin B12 requires tetrapyrrolic structural framework. This framework is created by the enzymes *deaminase* and *cosynthetase.* Tetrapyrrolic structural framework is responsible to transform aminolevulinic acid *via* porphobilinogen and hydroxymethylbilane to uroporphyrinogen III. The uroporphyrinogen III is the first macrocyclic intermediate common to haem, chlorophyll, sirohaem and B12 itself. Until the genetically-engineered strain of *Pseudomonas denitrificans* was used, eight of the genes involved in the biosynthesis of the vitamin had been over expressed, and the complete sequence of methylation and other steps could be determined, thus fully establishing all the intermediates in the pathway [37].

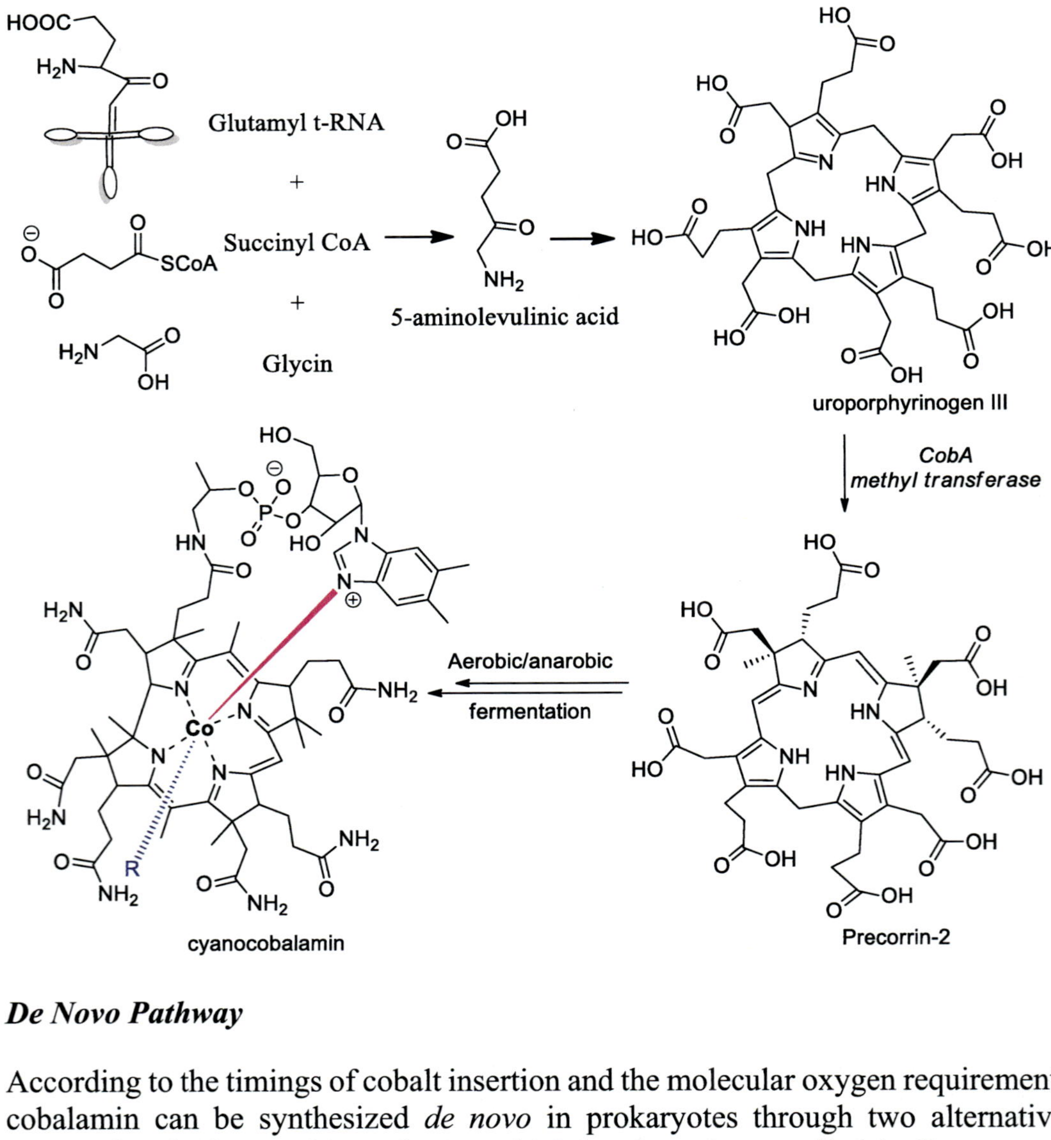

De Novo Pathway

According to the timings of cobalt insertion and the molecular oxygen requirement, cobalamin can be synthesized *de novo* in prokaryotes through two alternative routes. One is the aerobic pathway, which has been best studied in *Paracoccus denitrificans*, and second is the anaerobic pathway, in which *S. typhimurium*, *Bacillus megaterium*, and *P. shermanii* are used. These differ in terms of cobalt chelation and oxygen requirements.

Industrial Process

Streptomyces griseus was the commercial source of vitamin B12 for many years. The species *Pseudomonas denitrificans* and *Propionibacterium freudenreichii subsp. shermanii* are commonly used today for the industrial production of B12 [47b]. Rhone-Poulenc improved yield *via* genetic engineering *P. denitrificans*. At an early stage, Aventis Company used to produce vitamin B12, later merged to Sanofi-Aventis, and currently, Sanofi division is producing the same. At present, the French Sanofi-Aventis and three Chinese companies are producing vitamin B12 and till 2008 the total amount produced by these four company was 35,000 kg [38].

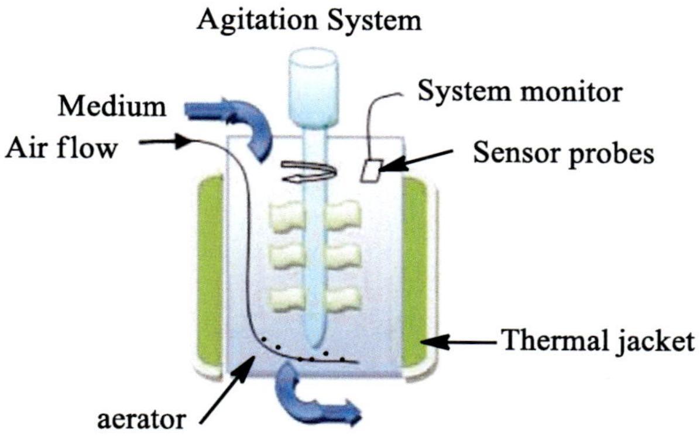

Fig. (2). Schematic presentation of industrial B12 production.

VITAMIN C (ASCORBIC ACID)

L-Ascorbic acid is the commonly used chemical name of vitamin C. This water soluble vitamin is essential for humans, non-human primates and a few other mammals. Vitamin C is related to the common disease of sailors and navies, namely scurvy with symptoms such as bleeding of mucous membranes, anaemia and ultimately death.Ascorbic acid participates in several biological processes *via* redox mechanism and is thereby used as an antioxidant. It is useful for the biosynthesis of collagen, the most abundant protein in the human body. For this reason, it is widely used as additives in cosmetics. Vitamin C also helps the body against carcinogenic nitrosamines and free radicals.

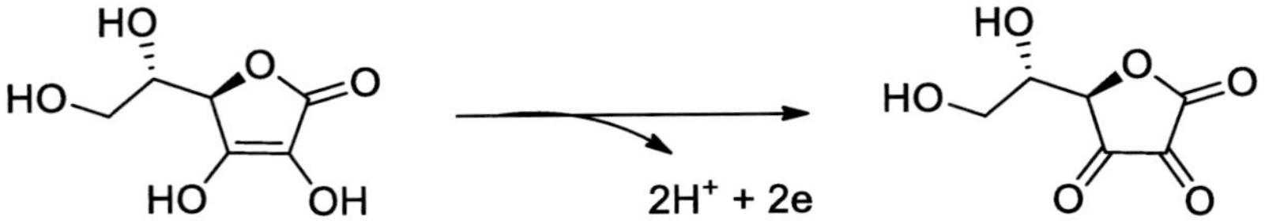

L-ascorbic acid Dehydroascorbic acid

In 1928, Ascorbic acid was ifrst isolated by Albert Szen□Gyørgyi from adrenal glands and named as hexuronic acid. Later, Charles Glen King confirmed that hexuronic acid is actually Ascorbic acid, whose structure was further confirmed by Norman Haworth in 1933. Tadeus Reichstein first developed the commercial synthesis of Ascorbic acid in bulk and still now this chemical and bacterial fermentation sequence is used today to produce vitamin C. In the early1970s, a two-step microbial fermentation process was developed in China which requires not only less chemicals and energy but also low investment in production equipment in comparison to the Reichstein process. Till 2015, using this process, China manufactured more than 80% of vitamin C in the world market.

Industrial Production of Vitamin C

Reichstein-Grussner Synthesis

Reichstein process is a combination of chemical and bacterial fermentation sequence for the production of vitamin C. Submerged bioreactor fermentation process is useful for this reaction. D-Glucose is first converted to D-sorbitol [48a]. Then, oxidation of D-sorbitol to L-sorbose is carried out initially by *Gluconobacter spp.* Currently, *Gluconobacter oxydans* or *Acetobacter suboxydans*, *sorbitol dehydro-genase* are being used for high conversion rate. This is completed almost after 24 hours at 30-35 °C temperature. Sorbose by a couple of chemical reactions can be finally converted to L-ascorbic acid. In the method by Reichstein-Grussner, 100 g of ascorbic acid is produced from 200 g of glucose. Hoffman□La Roche was the □rst pharmaceutical company which bought the Reichstein process patent for mass production of vitamin C under the brand name Redoxon® [15].

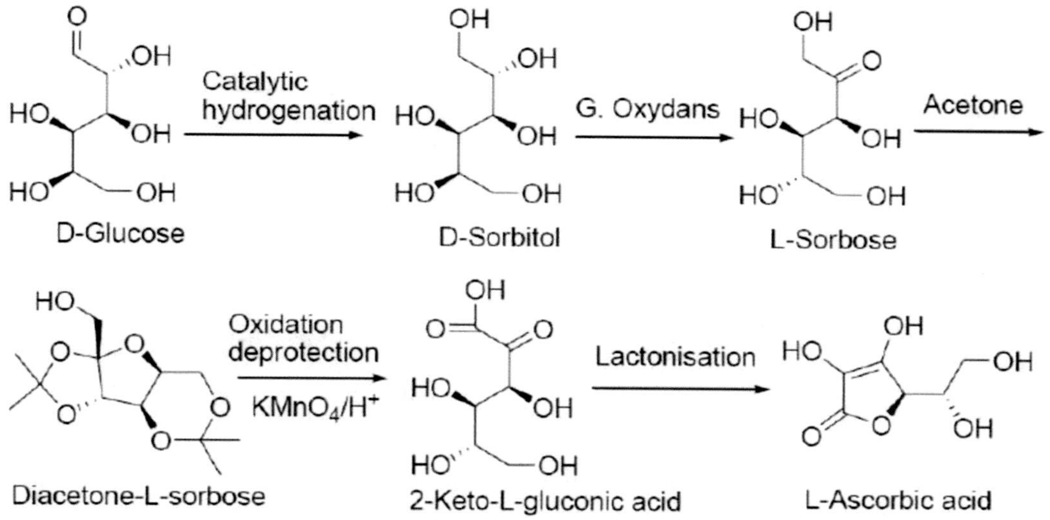

Two Step Fermentation Process

Initially, D-glucose is hydrogenated to D-sorbitol. The two-step fermentation process is very common. This process is superior to Reichstein-Grussner methods for low investment in production equipment and fewer chemicals and energy [48b].

1st Step: In the first step of fermentation, D-sorbitol is oxidized into L-sorbose by *G. oxydans*. This takes about 24h and results in a high concentration of L-sorbose (25–28%, w/v).

Substrate concentration	20–25%
Fermentation periods	18–24h
Productivity	12–13g/l/h
Temperature	32 °C
pH	natural
Oxygen transfer rate	300–500mmol/l/h

2nd Step: In the second step, 2-Keto-L-gulonic acid(2-KLG) is then produced from *L-sorbose* by a mixed culture of *K. vulgare* and *Bacillus sp*. This takes about 40-

70h with a lower product concentration (8–10%, w/v). This clearly indicates the low productivity and conversion rate of this process. It is also possible to involve *Bacillus megaterium* for converting L-sorbose to 2-keto-L- gluconic acids. Latter, by chemical reactions, 2-KLG is converted to ascorbic acid.

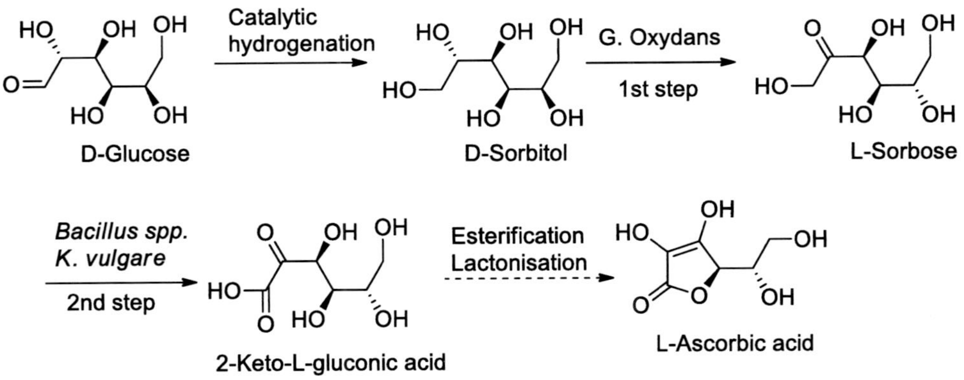

Substrate concentration	10mg/mL
Fermentation periods	40-65h
Productivity	90–110g/l
Temperature	29°C
pH	7.0
Oxygen transfer rate	100mmol/l/h

On the other hand, Biotechnologists have been successful in cloning and expressing the gene for 2,5-diketogluconic acid reductase of *Corynebacterium* sp. into *Erwinia herbicola*. By doing this, the two-step fermentation process has been reduced to one. The genetically engineered Erwinia cells were able to convert D-glucose directly to 2-keto-L-gluconic acid.

This is certainly advantageous since the metabolic capabilities of two different microorganisms (*Pseudomonas striata* and *G.oxydans*) could be combined into one organism. However, the yield of ascorbic acid by the hybrid strain was very low. Scientists are now trying to alter certain amino acids in 2-5 diketogluconic acid reductase and increase the catalytic activity of this enzyme. By optimisation, the conversion rate of L-sorbose to 2-keto-L-gluconic aid (2-KLG) of this co-culture system has been enhanced to 90–92%.

Chemically, 2-KLG is converted into L-ascorbic acid by acid transformation method. But alkali transformation method is widely used by the Chinese chemical companies due to the simple operation process and mild reaction conditions.

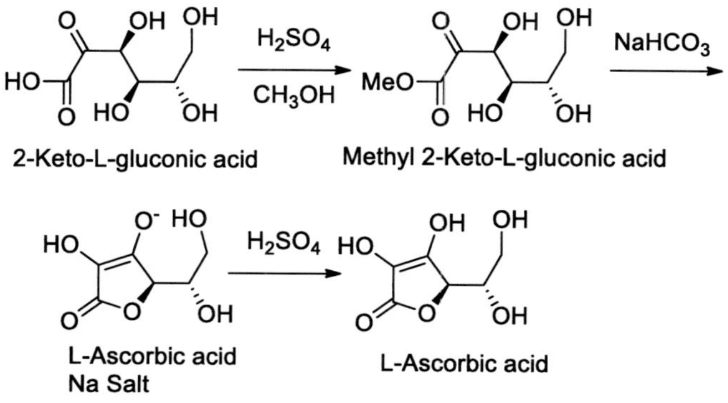

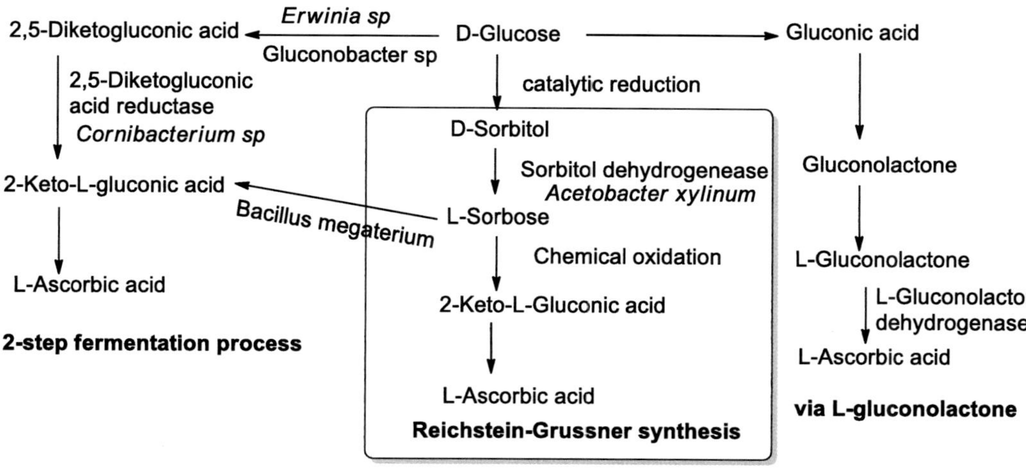

Commercial production of vitamin C

Yeast based stain *e.g. saccharomyces cerevisiae* can also produce L-ascorbic acid intracellularly when incubated with L-galactose. Antioxidant like carotene, L-ascorbic acid and vitamin E are simultaneously produced by *euglena gracilis* Z.

LIST OF ABBREVIATIONS

AI: **A**ctive **I**ngredient

ADME: **A**bsorption, **D**istribution, **M**etabolism, and **E**limination)

API: **A**ctive **P**harmaceutical **I**ngredient

DMPK: **D**rug **M**etabolism and **P**harmaco-**K**inetics

PD: **P**harmaco-**D**ynamics

PK: **P**harmaco-**K**inetics

COX: **C**yclooxygenase

ED_{50}: **E**ffective **D**ose **F**ifty

FDA: **F**ood and **D**rug **A**dministration

IC_{50}: **I**nhibitory **C**oncentration **F**ifty

LD_{50}: **L**ethal **D**ose **F**ifty

NSAID: **N**on-**S**teroidal **A**nti-**I**nflammatory **D**rugs

NDA: **N**ew **D**rug **A**pplication

SAR: **S**tructure-**A**ctivity-**R**elationship

APAP: N-**A**cetyl-**P**ara-**A**mino-**P**henol

SA: **S**alicylic **A**cid

ASA: **A**cetyl-**S**alicylic **A**cid

PG: **P**rosta-**G**landin

DMAP:4-N,N-**D**i-**M**ethyl-**A**mino-**P**yridine

DHF: **D**i-**H**ydro-**F**olic acid

GDN: 1,3-**G**lyceryl **D**i-**N**itrate

AZT: **Az**ido-**T**hymidine

ZDV: **Z**i-**D**o-**V**udine

AIDS: **A**cquired **I**mmune **D**eficiency **S**yndrome

HIV: **H**uman **I**mmunodeficiency **V**irus

RNA: **R**ibo-**N**ucleic **A**cid

DNA: **D**eoxy-**R**ibonucleic **A**cid

DDS: **D**iamino-**D**iphenyl **S**ulfone

DEAD:

CYP: **C**ytochrome **P**

NAT: **N**-**A**cetyl-**T**ransferase

HWE: **H**orner–**W**adsworth–**E**mmons

DIBAL: **Di**-**I**so-**B**utyl**al**uminium

TBDMS: **T**ert-**B**utyl-**Di**-**M**ethyl-**S**ilyl

DIAD: **Di**-**I**sopropyl **A**zo-**D**icarboxylate

HMDS: **H**exa-**M**ethyl-**Di**-**S**ilazane

TFA: **T**ri-**F**luoromethanesulfonic **A**cid

DMF: **D**i-**M**ethyl-**F**ormamide

THF: **T**etra-**H**ydro-**F**uran

NRTI: **N**ucleoside **R**everse-**T**ranscriptase **I**nhibitor

TNT: **T**ri-**N**itro-**T**oluene

GABA: **G**amma-**A**mino-**B**utyric **A**cid

FGA: **F**unctional **G**roup **A**ddition

FGI: **F**unctional **G**roup **I**nterconversion

ATP: **A**denosine **T**ri-**P**hosphate

DGGE: **D**enaturing **G**radient **G**el **E**lectrophoresis

LAB: **L**actic **A**cid **B**acteria

PCR: **P**olymerase **C**hain **R**eaction

ETC: **E**lectron **T**ransport **C**hain

NADH: **N**icotinamide **A**denine **D**inucleotide **H**ydrogen

$FADH_2$: **F**lavin **A**denine **D**inucleotide **H**ydrogen

GTP: **G**uanosine **T**ri-**P**hosphate

6-APA: 6-**A**mino-**P**enicillanic **A**cid

7-ACA: 7-**A**mino-**C**ephalosporanic **A**cid

DAO/ DAAO:D-**A**mino **A**cid **O**xidase

GLA : **Gl**utaryl-**A**cylase

2-KLG: 2-**K**eto-**L**-**G**ulonic acid

ALA: **Ala**nine

CPEC: **C**ircular **P**olymerase **E**xtension **C**loning

LCR : **L**ocus **C**ontrol **R**egion

FAD: **F**lavin **A**denine **D**inucleotide

FMN: **F**lavin **M**ono-**N**ucleotide

NMDA: **N**-**M**ethyl-**D**-**A**spartate

SLIC: **S**equence- and **L**igation-**I**ndependent **C**loning

REFERENCES

[1] Newman, D. J.; Cragg, G. M. Natural products as sources of new drugs over the last 25 years *J. Nat. Prod.*, **2007**, *70*, 461–477.

[2] Roger, M. J.; Reigosa, M. J.; Pedrol, N.; González, L. *Allelopathy: a physiological process with ecological implications*, Springer, 1st Eds.; Springer Netherlands, **2006.**

[3] Patrick, G. L. Introduction to Medicinal Chemistry, Oxford University Press, UK, 2013.

[4] (a) Singh, H.; Kapoor, V. K. Medicinal and Pharmaceutical Chemistry, Vallabh Prakashan, Pitampura, New Delhi, 2012. (b) Smith, Janice G. Organic Chemistry; McGraw Hill Companies, 2011; pp. 642-643.

[5] Foye, W. O.; Lemke, T. L.; William, D. A. Principles of Medicinal Chemistry, 4th Ed., B. I. Waverly Pvt. Ltd. New Delhi, 1995.

[6] The Textbook of Pharmaceutical Medicine Edited by J. P. Griffin 6th ed. Wiley-Blackwell, Singapore, 2009.

[7] Clayden, J.; Greeves, N.; Warren, S. Organic Chemistry, Second edition, Oxford University Press 2012.

[8] Warren, J. Drug discovery: lessons from evolution *Br. J. Clin. Pharmacol.*, **2011**, *71*, 497–503.

[9] https://druginfo.nlm.nih.gov/drugportal/

[10] Nocent, M.; Bertocchi, L.; Espitalier, F.; Baron, M.; Couarraze, G. Definition of a solvent system for spherical crystallization of salbutamol sulfate by quasi - emulsion solvent diffusion (qesd) method. *J. Pharm. Sci.* **2001**, *90*, 1620-1627.

[11] Chang, B. S.; Hershenson, S. Practical approaches to protein formulation development. In Rationale Design of stable protein formulations-theory and practice, Carpente, J. F.; Manning, M. C. Eds. Kluwer Academic/Plenum publishers, New York, **2002,** pp. 1-25.

[12] Hughes, J. P.; Rees, S.; Kalindjian, S. B.; Philpott, K. L. Principles of early drug discovery *Br J. Pharmacol.,* **2011**, *162*, 1239–1249.

[13] https://www.drugbank.ca/drugs/

[14] https://www.drugs.com/drug_information.html

[15] http://www.drugsupdate.com/

[16] Aspirin: (a) Randall, J. *The Synthesis and Analysis of Aspirin.* In *Advanced Chemistry with Vernier* **2013;** (b) Palleros, D. R. *Experimental organic chemistry. New York: John Wiley & Sons.* **2000,** p. 494; (c) Montes, I.; Sanabria, D.; García, M.; Castro, J.; Fajardo, J. A Greener Approach to Aspirin Synthesis Using Microwave Irradiation *J. Chem. Edu.*, **2006**, *83*, 628-631.

[17] https://www.drugfuture.com

[18] Ibuprofen: (a) Ibanez, J. G. *The Minimization and Prevention of Pollution*; Green Chemistry. In Environmental Chemistry. Springer, New York, NY, **2007;** (b) Faigl, F.; Schlosser, M. A one-pot synthesis of ibuprofene involving three consecutive steps of superbase metalation *Tetrahedron Lett.*, **1991**, *32*, 3369-3370; (c) Agee, B. M.; Mullins, G.; Swartling, D. J. Friedel–Crafts Acylation Using Solar Irradiation *Sustain Chem Process* **2016,** *4*, 8; (d) Cleij, M. *et al.* Microbiological Transformations 43. Epoxide Hydrolases as Tools for the Synthesis of Enantiopure α-Methylstyrene Oxides: A New and Efficient Synthesis of (S)-Ibuprofen *J. Org. Chem.,* **1999,** *64*, 5029.

[19] Paracetamol: (a) Ellis, F. *Paracetamol: a curriculum resource. Cambridge: Royal Society of Chemistry.* **2002;** (b) Joncour, R.; Duguet, N.; Métay, E.; Ferreira, A.; Lemaire, M. Amidation of phenol derivatives: a direct synthesis of paracetamol (acetaminophen) from hydroquinone *Green Chem.* **2014,** *16*, 2997-3002; (c) Friderichs, E.; Christoph, T.; Buschmann, H. *Analgesics and Antipyretics, Ullmann's Encyclopedia of Industrial Chemistry, Weinheim: Wiley-VCH.* 2011, (d) Ghiaci, M.; Aghaei, H.; Oroojeni, M.; Aghabarari, B.; Rives, V.; Vicente, M. A.; Sobrados, I.; Sanz, J. Synthesis of paracetamol by liquid phase Beckmann rearrangement of 4-hydroxyacetophenone oxime over H3PO4/Al-MCM-41. *Catal. Commun.*, 2009, 10, 1486-1492.

[20] Chloroquine: (a) Nsumiwa, S.; Kuter, D.; Wittlin, S.; Chibale, K.; Egan, T. J. Structure–activity relationships for ferriprotoporphyrin IX association and β-hematin inhibition by 4-aminoquinolines using experimental and ab initio methods *Bioorg. Med. Chem.,* **2013**, *21*, 3738-3748; (b) Johnson, W. S.; Buell, B. G. A New Synthesis of Chloroquine *J. Am. Chem. Soc.,* **1952**, *74*, 4513-4516; (c) Gould–Jacobs Reaction. Comprehensive Organic Name Reactions and Reagents. **276**. 2010. pp. 1252–1255; (d) Wang, Z. Gould-Jacobs Reaction. Comprehensive Organic Name Reactions and

Samir Kumar Mandal and Rebeca Ghanta

Reagents. **2010,** John Wiley & Sons, Inc. (e) Nzila, A. Inhibitors of de novo folate enzymes in Plasmodium falciparum *Drug Discov. Today* **2006**, *11*, 939-944;

[21] Premaquin: Kaur, H.; Machado, M.; Kock, C.; Smith, P.; Chibale, K.; Prudêncio, M.; Singh, K. Primaquine–pyrimidine hybrids: Synthesis and dual-stage antiplasmodial activity *Eur. J. Med. Chem.,* **2015**, *101*, 266-273.

[22] Norfloxacin: (a) Patent US4146719 - Piperazinyl derivatives of quinoline carboxylic acids - Google Patents"; (b) Vardanyan, R. S.; Hruby, V. J. Antimicrobial Drugs, In Synthesis of Essential Drugs, **2006**, pp 499-523.

[23] Chloramphenicol: (a) Park, J. N.; Ko, S. Y.; Koh, H. Y. Synthetic applications of the cyclic iminocarbonate rearrangement Enantioselective syntheses of chloramphenicol and 4-epi-cytoxazone *Tetrahedron Lett.,* **2000**, *41*, 5553-5556; (b) Long, L. M.; Troutman, H. D. Chloramphenicol (Chloromycetin). VI. A Synthetic Approach *J. Am. Chem. Soc.,* **1949**, *71*, 2469–2472. (c) Wu, G.-Z.; Tormos, W. I. Asymmetric process for preparing florfenicol, thiamphenicol chloramphenicol and oxazoline intermediates **1992**, U.S. Patent US5352832; (d) Dinos, G. P.; Athanassopoulos, C. M.; Missiri, D. A.; Giannopoulou, P. C.; Vlachogiannis, I. A.; Papadopoulos, G. E.; Papaioannou, D.; Kalpaxis, D. L. Chloramphenicol Derivatives as Antibacterial and Anticancer Agents: Historic Problems and Current Solutions *Antibiotics*, **2016**, *5*, 20.

[24] Sulphacetamide : (a) Crossley, M. L.; Northey, E. H.; Hultquist, M. E. Sulfanilamide Derivatives. IV. N^1,N^4-Diacylsulfanilamides and N^1-Acylsulfanilamides *J. Am. Chem. Soc.,* **1939,** *61,* 2950–2955; (b) Brown, G. M. The biosynthesis of folic acid. II. Inhibition by sulfonamides *J. Biol. Chem.,* **1962,** *237*, 536-540.

[25] Trimethoprim: (a) Zinner, S. H.; Mayer, K. H. Sulfonamides and Trimethoprim. In Principles and Practice of Infectious Diseases, G. L. Mandell, G. E. Douglas, and R. Bennett's (Eighth Edition), Elsevier, **2015,** pp 475-486; (b) Takagishi, Y.; Ohsuga, K.; Ohama, S. Suppository containing sulfamethoxazole/trimethoprim complex and process for preparing the same **1975**, U.S. Patent US4461765.

[26] Fluconazole: (a) Szeto, J.; Vu, V-A.; Malerich, J. P. Multi-step continuous flow synthesis of fluconazole *J. Flow. Chem.*, **2019**, *9*, 35-42; (b) Owoyemi, B. C. D.; da Silva, C. C. P.; Souza, M. S.; Diniz, L. F.; Ellena, J.; Carneiro, R. L. Fluconazole: Synthesis and Structural Characterization of Four New Pharmaceutical Cocrystal Forms *Cryst. Growth Des.,* **2019**, *19*, 648-657; (c) Joseph-Horne, T.; Hollomon, D. W. Molecular mechanisms of azole resistance in fungi *FEMS Microbiol Lett.* **1997**, *149*, 141-149; (d) Houšť, J.; Jaroslav Spížek, J.; Havlíček, V. Antifungal Drugs *Metabolites*, **2020**, *10*, 106.

[27] Phenobarbital: (a) Nantachit, K.; Santiarworn, D.; Kumdech, N.; Luecha, N. Synthesis of Phenobarbital, An anticonvulsant Drug *CMU. J. Nat. Sci.,* **2007**, *6*, 49-56; (b) Lednicer, D.; Mitscher, L. A. The Organic Chemistry of Drug Synthesis, 2, *New York: John Wiley & Sons.* **1980,** p 304, 365; (c) Sun, T.; Watson, S.; Manchanda, R. U.S. Patent US20100035904, (d) Marc, I. N.; Haverstraw, N.; Bilter, W. Preparation of Phenobarbital **1944**, US2358072.

[28] Diazepam : (a) Gates, M. New Synthesis of Diazepam *J. Org. Chem.,* **1980**, *45*, 1675-1681; (b) Massah, A. R.; Gharaghani, S.; Lordejani, H. A.; Asakere, N. *Med. Chem. Res.,* New and mild method for the synthesis of alprazolam and diazepam and computational study of their binding mode to GABAA receptor *Med. Chem. Res.* **2016**, *25*, 1538–1550; (c) Orlov, V. Y.; Kotov, A. D.; Bystryakova, E. B.; Kopeikin, V. V.; Mironov, G. S. *Russ. J. Org. Chem.,* **1994**, *30*, 1481–1484; (d) Lednicer, D.; Mitscher, L. A. The Organic Chemistry of Drug Synthesis, *2, New York: John Wiley & Sons.* **1980,** *p 304, 365;* (e) Blancafort, P.; Serradell, M. N.; Castaor, J. *Drugs Fut.*, **1981**, *6*, 774; (f) Ozlen, G, Alessio, I; Daniela, V;, Andrea, S;. Supuran, T.; Claudiu Innocenti, A. 3-Phenyl-1H-Indole-5-Sulfonamides: Structure-Based Drug Design of a Promising Class of Carbonic Anhydrase Inhibitors *Curr. Pharm. Des.,* **2010**, *16*, 3317–3326; (g) Alois, F.; Achim, H.; Günter, S. *Org. Synth.,* **1999**, *76*, 142.

[29] Nitroglycerin : (a) Ferreira, J. C.; Mochly-Rosen, D. Nitroglycerin use in myocardial infarction patients *Circ. J.* **2012**,*76*, 15-21; (b) Fan, Q.; Chen, L.; Cheng, S.; Li, F.; Lau, W. B.; Wang, L.; Liu, J. Oxidative medicine and cellular longevity. 2014. 376515. 10.1155/2014/376515.

[30] Dapsone: (a) Ferry, C. W.; Buck, J. S.; Baltzly, R. *Org. Synth.* **1942**, *22*, 31, DOI: 10.15227/orgsyn.022.0031; (b) Weijiard, J.; Messerly, J. P. Dapsone **1945**, U.S. Patent 2,385,899; (c) Fromm, E.; Wittmann, Derivate des p-Nitrothiophenols *J. Ber.* **1908**, *41*, 2264-2273; (d) Zhu, Y. I.; Stiller, M. J. Dapsone and sulfones in dermatology: overview and update *J. Am. Acad. Dermatol.* **2001**, *45*, 420-434; (e) Oliveira, F. R.; Pessoa, M. C.; Albuquerque, R. F. V.; Schalcher, T. R.;

Monteiro, M. C. Clinical Applications and Methemoglobinemia Induced by Dapsone *J. Braz. Chem. Soc.*, **2014**, *25*, 1770-1779.

[31] Acyclovir: (a) Izawa, K.; Shiragami, H. Practical syntheses of antiviral nucleosides *Pure & Appl. Chem.*, **1998**, *70*, 313-318; (b) Lednicer, D.; Mitscher, L. A. The Organic Chemistry of Drug Synthesis, 3, *New York: John Wiley & Sons.*, **1980,** p 230; (c) O'Brien, J. J.; Campoli-Richards, D. M. Acyclovir. An updated review of its antiviral activity, pharmacokinetic properties and therapeutic efficacy *Drugs* **1989**, *37*, 233-309. (d) Miller, W. H.; Miller, R. L. Phosphorylation of acyclovir diphosphate by cellular enzymes *Biochem. Pharmacol.*, **1982**, *31*, 3879-84. (e) Castanerr, J.; Hillier, K. *Drugs Fut.* **1978**, *3*, 788; (f) Schaeffer, H. J. Acyclovir chemistry and spectrum of activity *Am. J. Med.*, **1982**, *73*, 4-6; (g) Schaeffer, H. J.; Beauchamp, L.; de Miranda, P.; Elion, G. B.; Bauer, D. J.; Collins, P. 9-(2-Hydroxyethoxymethyl)guanine activity against viruses of the herpes group *Nature*, **1978**, *272*, 583-585; (h) Gao, H.; Mitra, A. K. Synthesis of Acyclovir, Ganciclovir and Their Prodrugs: A Review *Synthesis*, **2000**, *3*, 329-351.

[32] AZT**:** (a) Gauthier, C.; Ramondenc, Y.; Plé, G. A novel synthesis of AZT *Tetrahedron* **2001**, *57*, 7513-7517; (b) Kenney, K. B.; Wring, S. A.; Carr, R. M.; Wells, G. N.; Dunn, J. A. Simultaneous determination of zidovudine and lamivudine in human serum using HPLC with tandem mass spectrometry *J. Pharm. Biomed. Sci.*, **2000**, *22*, 967-983; (c) Saunders, J. *Top Drugs*, Oxford Science Publications, **2000**; (d) Czernecki, S.; Valéry, J-M. An Efficient Synthesis of 3′-Azido-3′-deoxythymidine (AZT) *Synthesis*, **1991**, 239-240; (e) Glinski, R. P.; Khan, M. S.; Kalamas, R. L.; Sporn, M. B. Nucleotide synthesis. IV. Phosphorylated 3'-amino-3'-deoxythymidine and 5'-amino-5'-deoxythymidine and derivatives *J. Org. Chem.* **1973**, *38*, 25, 4299-4305.

[33] Warren, S. Organic Synthesis the Disconnection Approach, John Wiley and Sons.

[34] Warren, S. Designing Organic Synthesis, Wiley India, 2009.

[35] Aerobic and Anaerobic fermentation**:** (a) Cooper, G. M. *The Cell: A Molecular Approach*. 2nd edition. Sunderland (MA): Sinauer Associates. **2000;** (b) Ciani, M.; Comitini, F.; Mannazzu, I. *Fermentation* In *Encyclopedia of Ecology*, **2013,** Vol 2, pp 310-321; (c) Saxena, S. *Applied Microbiology*, Springer India; (d) Pham, J. V.; Yilma, M. A.; Feliz, A., Majid, M. T.; Maffetone, N.; Walker, J. R.; Kim, E.; Cho, H. J.; Reynolds, J. M.; Song, M. C.; Park, S. R.; Yoon, Y. J. A Review of the Microbial Production of Bioactive Natural Products and Biologics. *Front. Microbiol.* **2019**, *10*, 1404. doi: 10.3389/fmicb.2019.01404. (e) Santos, M.S., Nogueira, M.A. & Hungria, M. Microbial inoculants: reviewing the past, discussing the present and previewing an outstanding future for the use of beneficial bacteria in agriculture. AMB Expr 9, 205 (2019). https://doi.org/10.1186/s13568-019-0932-0.

[36] Metzler, D. E. Biochemistry: The Chemical Reactions Of Living Cells Vols 1& 2, 2 Ed., Elsevier Acadeic Press.

[37] Nelson, D. L.; Cox, M. M.; Lehninger Principles of Biochemistry: International Edition, WH Freeman; 7th ed. 2017.

[38] https://www.sciencedirect.com/topics/engineering/microbial-process

[39] https://www.generalmicroscience.com/

[40] (a) Borresen, E. C., Henderson, A. J., Kumar, A., Weir, T. L., & Ryan, E. P. (2012). Fermented foods: patented approaches and formulations for nutritional supplementation and health promotion. Recent patents on food, nutrition & agriculture, 4(2), 134–140. https://doi.org/10.2174/2212798411204020134; (b) Tamang, J. P.; Cotter, P. D.; Endo, A.; Han, N. S.; Kort, R.; Liu, S. Q.; Mayo, B.; Westerik, N.; Hutkins, R. Fermented foods in a global age: East meets West, *Compr. Rev. Food Sci. Food Saf.*, **2020**, *19*, 184-217.

[41] Ethyl alcohol: (a) Walker, G. M.; Walker, R. S. K. Enhancing Yeast Alcoholic Fermentations In Advances in Applied Microbiology, Elsevier Inc., **2018,** Vol 105, pp 87-129; (b) Malakar, S.; Paul, S. K.; Pou, K. R. J. Biotechnological Interventions in Beverage Production, In The Science of Beverages Academic Press, **2020,** Vol. 19, pp 1-37.

[42] Citric acid: (a) Currie, J. N. The Citric Acid Fermentation Of *Aspergillus Niger J. Biol. Chem.*, **1917**, *31*, 15-37; (b) Show, P. L.; Oladele, K. O.; Siew, Q. Y.; Zakry, F. A. A.; Lan, J. C.-W.; Ling, T. C. Overview of citric acid production from *Aspergillus niger Front. Life Sci.*, **2015**, 8, 271-283; (c) Vandenberghe, L. P.; Soccol, C. R.; Pandey, A.; Lebeault, J-M. Microbial production of citric acid *Braz. Arch. Biol. Technol.*, **1999**, *42*, 263–276 (d) Soccol, C.R., Vandenberghe, L.P.S., Rodrigues, C. and Pandey, A. New Perspectives for Citric Acid Production and Applications. *Food Technology and Biotechnology*, **2006**, *44*, 141-149; (e) Gupta, J.; Heding, L.; Jorgensen, O. Effect of sugars, hydrogen ion concentration and ammonium nitrate on the formation of citric acid by *Aspergillus Niger Acta*

Microbiol. Acad. Sci. Hung., **1975**, *23*, 63–67; (f) del Campo, G.; Berregi, I.; Caracena, R.; Santos. J. Quantitative analysis of malic and citric acids in fruit juices using proton nuclear magnetic resonance spectroscopy *Anal. Chim. Acta.*, **2006,** *556*, 462–468; (g) Moyer, A. J. Effect of alcohols on the mycological production of citric acid in surface and submerged culture. I. Nature of the alcohol effect. *J. App. Microbio.* **1953,** *1*, 1-7; (h) Li, C.; Xu, D.; Zhao, M.; Sun, L.; Wang, Y. Production optimization, purification, and characterization of a novel acid protease from a fusant by *Aspergillus Oryzae* and *Aspergillus Niger Eur. Food Res. Technol.*, **2014**, *238*, 905-917.

[43] Antibiotic (Penicillin, Cephalosporin, Chloromycetin, Streptomycin): (a) Gutiérrez, S.; Casqueiro, J.; Martín, J. F. *Production of Antibiotics* In Biotechnology – Vol. V, UNESCO- Encyclopedia of Life Support Systems, pp 126-151, (b) Metzler, D. E. *Biochemistry: The Chemical Reactions of Living Cells*, Academic Press, **2003,** Vol 1-2, 2 edition; (c) Barredo, J.-L. *Microbial Processes and Products,* Humana Press, **2005;** (d) Reynolds, D. M.; Schatz, A.; Waksman, S. A. Grisein, a new antibiotic produced by a strain of *Streptomyces griseus Proc. Soc. Exptl. Biol. Med.*, **1947**, *64*, 50-54; (e) Johnstone, D. B.; Waksman, S. A. The production of streptomycin by Streptomyces bikiniensis. *J. Bacteriol.*, **1948**, *55*, 317-326; (f) Isogai, T.; Fukagawa, M.; Aramori, I.; Iwami, M.; Kojo, H.; Ono, T.; Ueda, Y.; Kohsaka, M.; Imanaka, H. Construction of a 7-Aminocephalosporanic Acid (7ACA) Biosynthetic Operon and Direct Production of 7ACA in Acremonium Chrysogenum *Nat. Biotechnol.*, **1991**, *9*, 188–191, https://doi.org/10.1038/nbt0291-188; (g) Grögera, H.; Pieper, M.; König, B.; Bayer, T.; Schleich, H. Industrial landmarks in the development of sustainable production processes for the β-lactam antibiotic key intermediate 7-aminocephalosporanic acid (7-ACA) *Sustain Chem Pharm.* **2017**, *5*, 72-79; (h) Chemical Aspects of Enzyme Biotechnology: Fundamentals, **1990**, edited by Thomas O. Baldwin, Frank M. Raushel, A. Ian Scott, Springer Science.

[44] Lysine: (a) Félix, F. K. do C.; Letti, L. A. J.; Pereira, G. V. de M.; Bonfim, P. G. B.; Soccol, V. T.; Soccol, C. R. L-lysine production improvement: a review of the state of the art and patent landscape focusing on strain development and fermentation technologies *Crit. Rev. Biotechnol.*, **2019,** *39*, 1031-1055; (b) Shah, A. H.; Hameed, A.; Khan, G. M. Fermentative Production of L-Lysine: Bacterial Fermentation-I *J. Med. Sci.*, **2002**, *2,* 152-157; (c) Anastassiadis, S. *Recent Patents on Biotechnology*, **2007**, *1*, 11-24.

[45] Glutamic acid: (a) Kanzaki, T.; Isobe, K.; Okazaki, H.; Motizuki, K.; Fukuda, H. l-Glutamic Acid Fermentation: Part I. Selection of an Oleic Acid-Requiring Mutant and its PropertiesPart II. The Production of l-Glutamic Acid by an Oleic Acid-Requiring Mutant *Agric. Biol. Chem.*, **1967,** *31*, 1307-1317**;** (b) Chattopadhyay, S. P.; Banerjee, A. K. Production of l-glutamic acid by aBacillus sP. *Folia Microbiol.*, **1978,** *23*, 469-480**; (c)** Miller, A. L. Therapeutic considerations of L-glutamine: a review of the literature *Altern. Med. Rev.* **1999**, *4*, 239-48.

[46] Vitamin B2: Ledesma-Amaro, R.; Serrano-Amatriain, C.; Jiménez, A.; Revuelta, J. L. Metabolic engineering of riboflavin production in Ashbya gossypii through pathway optimization *Microb. Cell Fact.*, **2015,** *14*, https://doi.org/10.1186/s12934-015-0354-x; (b) Revuelta, J. L.; Ledesma-Amaro, R.; Lozano-Martinez, P.; Díaz-Fernández, D.; Buey, R. M.; Jiménez, A. Bioproduction of riboflavin: a bright yellow history *J. Ind. Microbiol. Biotechnol.* **2017**, *44*, 659–665.

[47] Vitamin B12: (a) Yamada, K. Cobalt: its role in health and disease *Met. Ions Life Sci.*, **2013**, *13*, 295–320; (b) Heinzle, E.; Biwer, A. P.; Cooney, C. L. *Development of Sustainable Bioprocesses: Modeling and Assessment,* **2006,** Wiley**.** (c) Chae, S.A.; Kim, H.-S.; Lee, J.H.; Yun, D.H.; Chon, J.; Yoo, M.C.; Yun, Y.; Yoo, S.D.; Kim, D.H.; Lee, S.A.; Chung, S.J.; Soh, Y.; Won, C.W. Impact of Vitamin B12 Insufficiency on Sarcopenia in Community-Dwelling Older Korean Adults. *Int. J. Environ. Res. Public Health* **2021**, *18*, 12433. https://doi.org/10.3390/ijerph182312433. (d) Hu, X.; Wei, X.; Ling, J.; Chen, J. Cobalt: An Essential Micronutrient for Plant Growth? *Front. Plant Sci.* **2021,** 12, 768523. doi: 10.3389/fpls.2021.768523 (e) Kräutler, B. Biochemistry of B12-cofactors in human metabolism. *Subcell Biochem.* **2012**, *56*, 323-346. doi: 10.1007/978-94-007-2199-9_17

[48] Vitamin C: (a) Yang, W.; Xu. H. *Industrial Fermentation of Vitamin C.* In *Industrial Biotechnology of Vitamins, Biopigments, and Antioxidants.* 1st Ed. E. J. Vandamme and J. L. Revuelta, Wiley-VCH Verlag GmbH & Co. KGaA, **2016,** pp 161-192. (b) Lim, S.M., Lau, M.S.L., Tiong, E.I.J. *et al.* Process design and economic studies of two-step fermentation for production of ascorbic acid. SN Appl. Sci. 2, 816 (2020). https://doi.org/10.1007/s42452-020-2604-8.

SUBJECT INDEX

A

Samir Kumar Mandal and Rebeca Ghanta

B

C

D

E

F

G

H

T

U

V

Y

Made in the USA
Las Vegas, NV
09 September 2025

266dd850-677a-4486-b21b-8929953f94a3R02